Nephrolithiasis - From Bench to Bedside

Edited by Mohammad Hammad Ather

Published in London, United Kingdom

Nephrolithiasis - From Bench to Bedside
http://dx.doi.org/10.5772/intechopen.101013
Edited by Mohammad Hammad Ather

Contributors
Farah Al-Mamoori, Talal Aburjai, Anshuman Singh, Milap Shah, B.M. Zeeshan Hameed, Ivan Thia, Matthew Chau, Mohammad Hammad Ather, Wajahat Aziz, Ahmad Bashir

First published in London, United Kingdom, 2023 by IntechOpen
IntechOpen is the global imprint of INTECHOPEN LIMITED, registered in England and Wales, registration number: 11086078, 5 Princes Gate Court, London, SW7 2QJ, United Kingdom

British Library Cataloguing-in-Publication Data
A catalogue record for this book is available from the British Library

Additional hard and PDF copies can be obtained from orders@intechopen.com

Nephrolithiasis - From Bench to Bedside
Edited by Mohammad Hammad Ather
p. cm.
Print ISBN 978-1-80355-111-1
Online ISBN 978-1-80355-112-8
eBook (PDF) ISBN 978-1-80355-113-5

Meet the editor

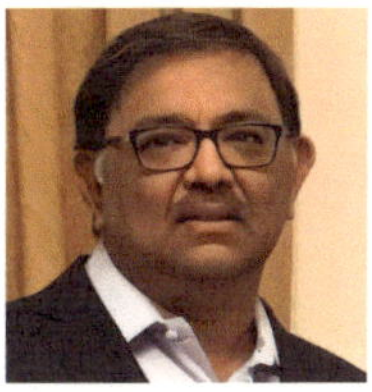

Professor Hammad Ather is a consultant urologist and endowed Professor of Urology at the Aga Khan University, Karachi. He is an editorial board member of many international urological journals. He is the author of more than 130 articles in international peer-reviewed journals and 10 book chapters. He has also edited four books. He is also an adviser and reviewer for more than two dozen international urological journals and for dissertations and theses at various universities. Prof. Ather was trained in Karachi and London. He has many fellowship attachments in Europe at Erasmus University Rotterdam, the Netherlands; Inselspital, University of Bern, Sweden; Katholique Universiteit Leuven, Belgium; and University College London. He served for over 5 years as the chair of the Ethics Review Committee (ERC) at Aga Khan University. He is a board member of the European Urolithiasis Society (EULIS), Asian Urological Surgery Training & Education Group (AUSTEG), and Urology Association of Asia (UAA) and president-elect of Pakistan Association of Urological Surgeons (PAUS).

Contents

Preface **IX**

Section 1
Management **1**

Chapter 1 **3**
Introductory Chapter: Complicated Urolithiasis
by Mohammad Hammad Ather

Chapter 2 **15**
Renal Tract Stones – Diagnosis and Management
by Ivan Thia and Matthew Chau

Chapter 3 **41**
Guideline Based Algorithmic Approach for the Management of Renal and Ureteric Calculi
by Anshuman Singh, Milap Shah and B.M. Zeeshan Hameed

Chapter 4 **57**
Perspective Chapter: Medicinal Plants for the Treatment of Nephrolithiasis
by Farah Al-Mamoori and Talal Aburjai

Section 2
Stone Prevention **67**

Chapter 5 **69**
Stone Prevention: Dietary Factors, Current Evidence, and Metabolic Workup
by Wajahat Aziz, Ahmad Bashir and Mohammad Hammad Ather

Preface

Changing epidemiology and global trends in the incidence of urolithiasis and rapid development both in our understanding of the pathophysiology of urolithiasis and the endourological revolution in its management merits publishing another treatise on this condition. Urolithiasis, once known to afflict people living in the Stone Belt, is fast becoming a global issue. This book addresses some of these developments. Authors from around the world discuss modern trends in the diagnosis, surgical management, and use of medicinal plants in treating kidney stones. Endourological management has significantly simplified the treatment of kidney and ureteral stones, but these procedures are still associated with significant morbidity and even mortality. The saying "prevention is better than cure" could not be more apt for kidney stone disease than any other condition. The book includes a chapter dedicated to stone prevention, analyzing the scientific merit of various dietary and pharmaceutical interventions.

Urolithiasis is at times complicated by other concurrent conditions related to the urinary tract or not related at all. Pregnancy and stone disease is one such example. Stones in the anomalous kidney and in the calyceal diverticula are conditions that can complicate the management of kidney stones. The introductory chapter examines these factors.

The book provides an impetus for further research and presents an overview of the current understanding of the management of kidney stones.

Mohammad Hammad Ather
Professor of Urology,
Aga Khan University,
Karachi, Pakistan

Section 1

Management

Chapter 1

Introductory Chapter: Complicated Urolithiasis

Mohammad Hammad Ather

1. Introduction

Urolithiasis management is simplified with the introduction of shock wave lithotripsy (SWL), in the 1980s, with the help of technological advances in endourology in the last quarter of the century. Stones are said to be "complicated" when they are associated with conditions which impact diagnosis and management. Stones in anomalous kidneys, stones following urinary diversion, stones formed/identified during pregnancy and stones in calyceal diverticulum are all considered to be complicated stones.

2. Kidney stones in pregnancy

The incidence of urolithiasis is increasing around the world. Urolithiasis is more common among men; however, the prevalence among women is increasing [1]. Around 7.1% women in the USA suffer from nephrolithiasis, and the incidence is on the rise [2]. Renal colic secondary to a kidney stone is the most common nonobstetric hospital admission diagnosis for pregnant women. The incidence of a symptomatic stones varies from 1 out of every 200–1500 pregnancies. Kidney stones in pregnancy are associated with significant complications including preterm labor and even delivery, premature rupture of the membranes, pregnancy loss, gestational hypertension which can lead to pre-eclampsia and urinary tract infections [3].

Women during pregnancy are more likely to form stones than otherwise [4]. Increased incidences of stones during pregnancy are often related to urinary stasis and collecting system dilation. It is a consequence of ureteral compression due to gravid uterus and progesterone-induced ureteral dilation. Besides anatomical factors, there are many biochemical changes favoring development of kidney stones. These include hypercalciuria and high urinary pH [5]. Imaging is not always successful in differentiating between obstruction and physiology. Majority of the stones are hydroxyapatite, mostly isolated and unilateral. The most common variety of stones formed during pregnancy is calcium phosphate (hydroxyapatite) [6]. The preponderance of hydroxyapatite stones is unclear; however, the probable cause is the pregnancy-related physiological alterations including increased calcium excretion and high urinary pH. The tendency to form stones continue to persist even after the pregnancy, during pregnancy second and third trimester and lasting until about 3 months following delivery [3].

Imaging is the cornerstone of diagnosis like in the nonpregnant population. Understandably ultrasound is the most frequently performed imaging. In various series, sensitivity of ultrasound in the detection of urolithiasis is highly variable. The reported sensitivity of ultrasound during pregnancy varies from 29 to 95% [7]. Ultrasound could be falsely negative in over two-third of the cases, as it relies mostly on secondary signs. Visualization of stones in the ureter is often difficult due to the gravid uterus and it relies on secondary signs, that is, hydroureter. Ureteral dilation during pregnancy is often due to a gravid uterus in over 90% of cases. The intrarenal resistive index (RI) estimation is an additional parameter that can improve the ability to differentiate obstruction from physiologic hydronephrosis. Mean value of 0.7 (45% sensitivity and 91% specificity) and difference between the two units of 0.06 (95% sensitivity and 100% specificity) is indicative of obstruction [8]. The other important Doppler ultrasound parameter frequently employed is the ureteral jet phenomenon. Both absence of ureteral jet and an elevated RI improves ultrasound's ability to diagnose obstruction from 56 to 72%. Transvaginal ultrasound is another important tool in the detection of distal ureteral stones [9]. In a study, it was observed that compared to transabdominal ultrasound, transvaginal ultrasound improves the ability to diagnose distal ureteral stones by threefold. The combination of transabdominal and transvaginal ultrasounds improve the ability to diagnose distal ureteral stones in 85% of the cases.

MRI scan is the second-line imaging if ultrasound fails to provide definitive answers. Both the AUA and EAU guidelines support this recommendation [7]. Noncontrast MR scans versus gadolinium enhanced studies (MR Urography) is still a contentious issue. However, American College of Obstetrics and gynecology (ACOG) recommends use of gadolinium contrast for scenarios where the benefit clearly outweighs the potential risks [10]. MRU without contrast (Single-shot turbo-spin echo) is reported to be 89% accurate in differentiating physiological hydronephrosis from obstruction secondary to urolithiasis. The overall positive predictive value of MR for ureteral stone is reported to be around 80% [11].

Noncontrast enhanced CT (CTKUB) is the gold standard in the evaluation of suspected uretero renal colic secondary to stone in both adult male and nonpregnant females and in children. However, radiation-induced nonstochastic (teratogenesis) or stochastic (carcinogenesis, mutagenesis) effects are a major concern. As a general principle, any imaging investigation resulting in an absorbed dose to the fetus of >0.5 mGy requires justification [11]. The teratogenic effects of fetal radiation exposure are cumulative with increasing dose. Potential fetal abnormalities include growth retardation, severe mental retardation, and microcephaly. Even the pregnancy loss can happen. The risk of fetal abnormalities is negligible at levels below 50 mSv. First two months of pregnancy and after 23rd week are safer periods. Current CT protocols particularly with low dose (<4 mSv) and ultralow dose CT (<1 mSv) are even safer. The current EAU guidelines recommend that ultrasound should be the preferred mode of imaging in pregnant women; MRI be used as second-line imaging and use low dose CT as a last option.

The contemporary management of acute kidney pain during pregnancy is by hydration, use of anti-emetics, and adequate pain control. Acetaminophen and if needed narcotics are safe for pain management. Spontaneous passage of stones is observed in 23-84% of cases [12]. Due to altered cell mediated immunity, up to 17% of women admitted with urolithiasis have accompanying pyelonephritis. Febrile infections secondary to obstructive uropathy are often observed due to altered cell mediated immunity. One in six women admitted for urolithiasis have pyelonephritis. Management is difficult due to limited choice in the use of medications. NSAIDs and codeine-containing medications for pain and fever and among antibiotics including penicillin, cephalosporins, and erythromycin are safer. Aminoglycosides, tetracycline, chloramphenicol, fluoroquinolones, and sulfa antibiotics, however, are contraindicated. Medical expulsive therapy use is 'off label' and belong to category B [13].

Interventional treatment is needed in about one in four to one in three pregnant women. Intervention is often indicated in cases of intractable pain, severe or progressive hydronephrosis, bilateral obstruction, or obstruction in a single functioning kidney, urosepsis secondary to obstructive uropathy. Women who develop obstetric complications like preterm labor or preeclampsia constitute failure of conservative treatment and mandate active intervention. Diversion using percutaneous nephrostomy (PCN) or insertion of double J stents are the most frequently performed [14]. There are pros and cons of both, whereas PCN is a shorter procedure under local anesthesia, it also facilitates subsequent PCNL (**Figure 1**) and is better in septic conditions, double J stents facilitates subsequent ureteroscopy, but often require a replacement in a matter of weeks to months due to higher incidence of encrustation and often require spinal anesthesia [15]. Ureteroscopy during pregnancy is associated with high success rates and should ideally be performed in the second trimester under either local or spinal anesthesia subject to ultrasound guidance. Fluoroscopy and general anesthesia should be avoided, particularly in the last trimester. PCNL and ESWL are associated with very high complication rates and should be avoided. ESWL is associated with miscarriage, congenital malformation, intrauterine growth retardation, placental disruption, and fetal demise [16], and therefore should not be performed.

In essence, urolithiasis during pregnancy is a challenge in both diagnosis and its management. Managing complex urolithiasis particularly with sepsis must be managed in a multidisciplinary setting with the active involvement of an obstetrician, radiologist, and urologist [17].

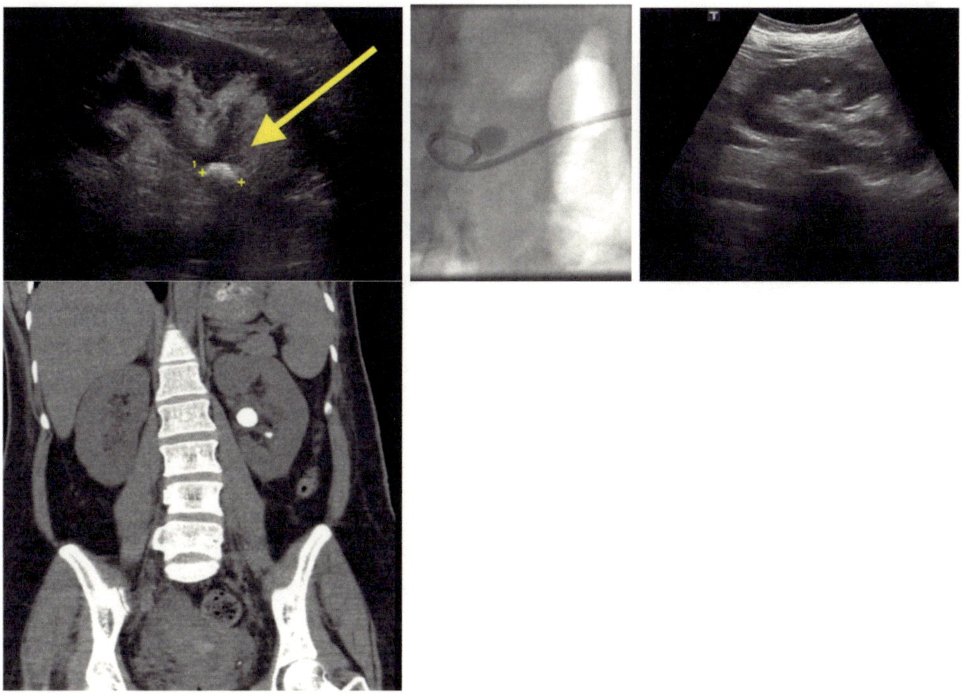

Figure 1.
A 27-year lady, 24 weeks pregnant presented to the emergency room with intractable pain, vomiting, and fever. Conservative management failed. Her ultrasound (A) showed hydrocalicosis and renal pelvic stone 15 mm. In view of failure of conservative treatment, a PCN was placed (B) and subsequent ultrasound (C) showed resolution of hydronephrosis, stone (arrow) and PCN. Postpartum CT (D) confirmed the presence of stone, and she underwent an unremarkable mPCNL.

3. Urolithiasis in urinary diversions

Removal of the urinary bladder for muscle invasive bladder cancer, requires urinary diversion. Urolithiasis following urinary diversion is a relatively frequent complication. Diversion increases the risk of urolithiasis due to anatomical factors such as kidney dysfunction and stasis, recurrent infections, metabolic abnormalities, and presence of foreign bodies, including mucous and exposed staple lines [18]. Stones can form in both the upper and lower urinary tract. In a series of over 1000 cystectomies and ileal conduit urinary diversion with a mean follow-up of 75 months, upper-tract urolithiasis was observed in 13.4%, whereas 4.5% developed stones in the conduit [19]. Similarly, stones are also formed in the reservoir as well in the upper tract in orthotopic neobladder formation. It is more frequently observed in stapled anastomosis compared to hand sewn [20].

Multiple factors play a role in increased incidence of urolithiasis with a urinary diversion. Metabolic abnormalities are more frequently observed following continent and orthotopic neobladder. Hyperchloremic metabolic acidosis, hypercalciuria, hyperoxaluria, and hypocitraturia are some common metabolic abnormalities in this

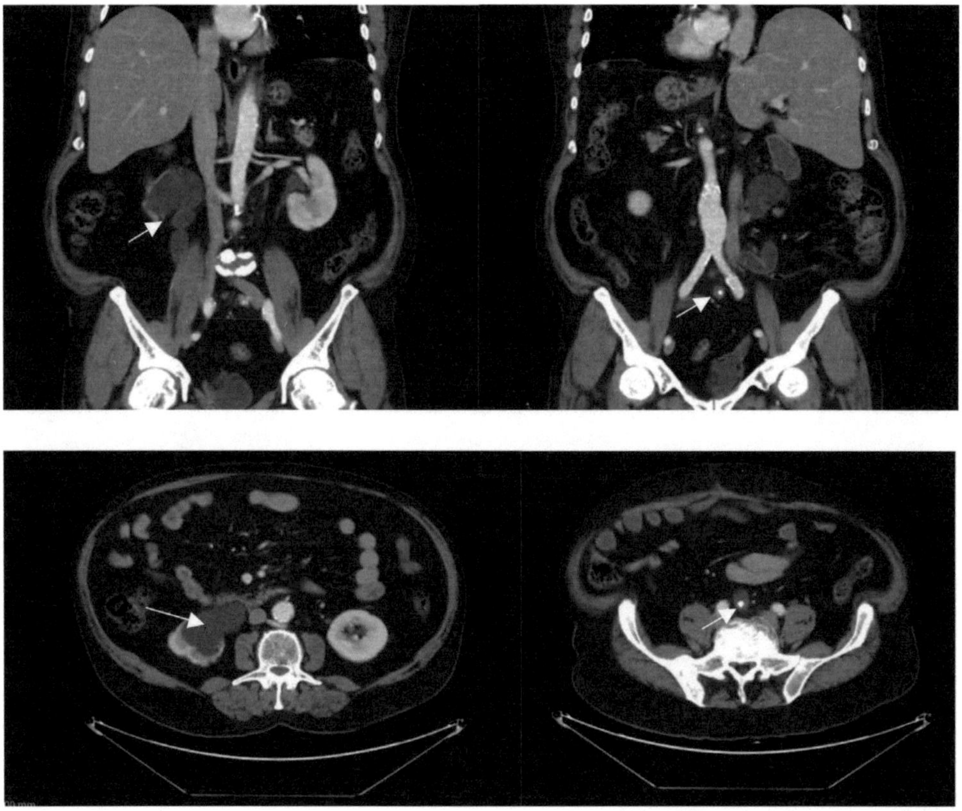

Figure 2.
A 68 years old had a radical cystectomy and orthotopic neobladder in 2015 for muscle invasive bladder cancer. He presented with left flank pain and hematuria 7 years after the surgery, work up indicated hydronephrosis (arrow a, c) right distal ureteral stone (a, d) slightly proximal to the uretero-ileal anastomosis. He was initially managed by oral dissolution therapy (potassium citrate) and medical expulsive treatment. Conservative treatment failed and was subsequently treated by rendezvous procedure with antegrade and retrograde flexible ureteroscopy.

cohort. The other changes like bone loss, recurrent infections, and development of CKD due to recurrent infections are major reasons for urinary hypercrystallization with stone formation. A cohort of 77 patients reported to have developed urolithiasis over 7 years of follow-up, Herzig et al. [21] noted that the most common stone composition was MAP stones in 63.5%, calcium phosphate stone in 25%, and only 11.5% were calcium oxalate stones (9.6% Wavellite and 1.9% Weddellite). Persistence of asymptomatic bacteriuria and urinary stasis following treatment of stones and infection results in high recurrence rate. Structural factors include presence of foreign bodies, urinary stasis, and mucus plugs providing nidus for recurrent urolithiasis. Foreign bodies include nonabsorbable sutures and staples, stents, and indwelling catheters. Urinary stasis results from inadequate emptying due to mucus and hypercontinence, uretero-intestinal anastomosis strictures, ureteric transposition (left-sided stones more common) [22], and stomal stenosis [23].

Interventional management of the stones involves flexible ureteroscopy (fURS) or combined ante and retrograde approaches, the rendezvous procedures. System is often dilated secondary to stones or obstruction; however, for nondilated systems, it is important to prestent the affected renal unit with an antegrade percutaneous tube (PCN) as well. This is needed for most complex stones and for easy maneuvering of the flexible instruments through difficult anatomy. For a nondilated system, ultrasound-guided puncturing on the stone, retrograde contrast study by placing a Foley's catheter with an inflated balloon and pushing contrast into the conduit for retrograde filling of the system is needed. If everything else fails, trauma protocol on table IVU with 2 mL of intravenous contrast may provide enough opacification for calyceal puncture. A careful inspection of the reservoir is important as foreign bodies (staples, sutures, etc.), stents mucus plugs forms a nidus for future recurrence. Most important is to achieve complete stone clearance and do medical treatment postoperatively to decrease recurrence. Infective stones are notoriously recurrent; therefore, 6–12 weeks of antibiotics are often recommended. For strictures and stenosis balloon dilation, stenting is recommended, and in certain situations, surgical revision of the uretero-intestinal anastomosis is recommended (**Figure 2**).

4. Urolithiasis in anomalous kidneys

The incidence of urolithiasis is higher in kidneys with anomalies of fusion, lie, or rotation [24].

Urolithiasis in anomalous kidneys pose special challenge due to differences in the lie rotation, and orientation of the calyces compared to an orthotropic kidney. Most common anomalous renal abnormalities include horseshoe kidney, ectopic pelvic kidney, and malrotated kidneys. Horseshoe kidney is the commonest of abnormalities. The anatomical anomaly causes fusion of lower pole which results in the abnormal position of UPJ, a high-placed UPJ, and malrotation and anterior displacement of the collecting system [25]. Preoperative work up should be meticulous to identify anatomical variations. CT urogram is often the study of choice. However, innovative meticulous planning uses artificial intelligence (AI) and 3D [26].

SWL, since its inception, due its non-invasive nature, became the treatment of choice. It is not suitable for most Kidney stones in anomalous kidneys due to location and even when appropriate, it is often associated with significant residual

Renal anomaly	Incidence	Anatomical variations
Horseshoe kidney	1 in 400 (live birth)	Abnormally placed UPJ High UPJ Anterior and malrotated calyx
Ectopic kidney	1 in 1000 (live birth)	Location and relationship with surrounding organs
Malrotated kidney	1 in 2000 (autopsy)	Variable orientation of renal pelvis, collecting system, and renal vessels
Calyceal diverticulum	Rare	Outpouchings from the collecting system, epithelial lining, muscular layer, and narrow channel

UPJ = Ureteropelvic junction.

Table 1.
Renal anomalies, incidence, and anatomical variations causing urolithiasis.

fragmentation and poor clearance. The stone clearance is reported to be under 70% in larger reported studies [14]. In a well-equipped endourology center, SWL is not the first choice in most anomalous kidney stones (**Table 1**).

Lim et al. [27] performed an interesting global study on the propensity score-matched pair analysis on data collected from 20 centers with urolithiasis in anomalous kidneys, Being treated with retrograde intrarenal surgery (RIRS) or mini PCNL (mPCNL). The treatment decision was made by the operating surgeon according to his preference and expertise. Authors concluded that both mPCNL and RIRS are safe and efficacious with mPCNL, demonstrating a higher stone free rate. Stones in anomalous kidneys are a complex medical condition and require expertise and availability of most endourological armamentarium. The treatment must be tailored according to individual needs of the patient. In patients with moderate-to-high stone burden, ectopic kidney's access to both RIRS and mPCNL is important. Endoscopic combined intra renal surgery (ECIRS) Often provides the necessary access to right calyx and do directed treatment (**Table 2**).

One of the major concerns when performing mPCNL on anomalous kidneys is the risk of bleeding. In a recent paper, Feng et al. [28] observed that Tranexamic acid may be a useful adjunct to prevent major bleeding. Technological developments in flexible ureteroscopy have made the RIRS as a first choice for most small-to-moderate size stones in the anomalous kidney. It is also indicated in situations where either SWL or mPCNL is not feasible or has failed (**Figure 3**).

Renal anomaly	mPCNL	RIRS	ECIRS	SWL
Horseshoe kidney	+++	++	+++	+
Ectopic kidney	+	+++	+	—
Malrotated kidney	+++ (for stones >2 cm)	+++ (for stones ≤2 cm)	+++	+
Calyceal diverticulum	++	++	+++	—

Level of recommendation = +; mPCNL = mini percutaneous nephrolithotomy; RIRS = Retrograde intrarenal surgery; SWL = Shock wave lithotripsy.

Table 2.
Pros and cons of various treatment options in renal anomalies with urolithiasis.

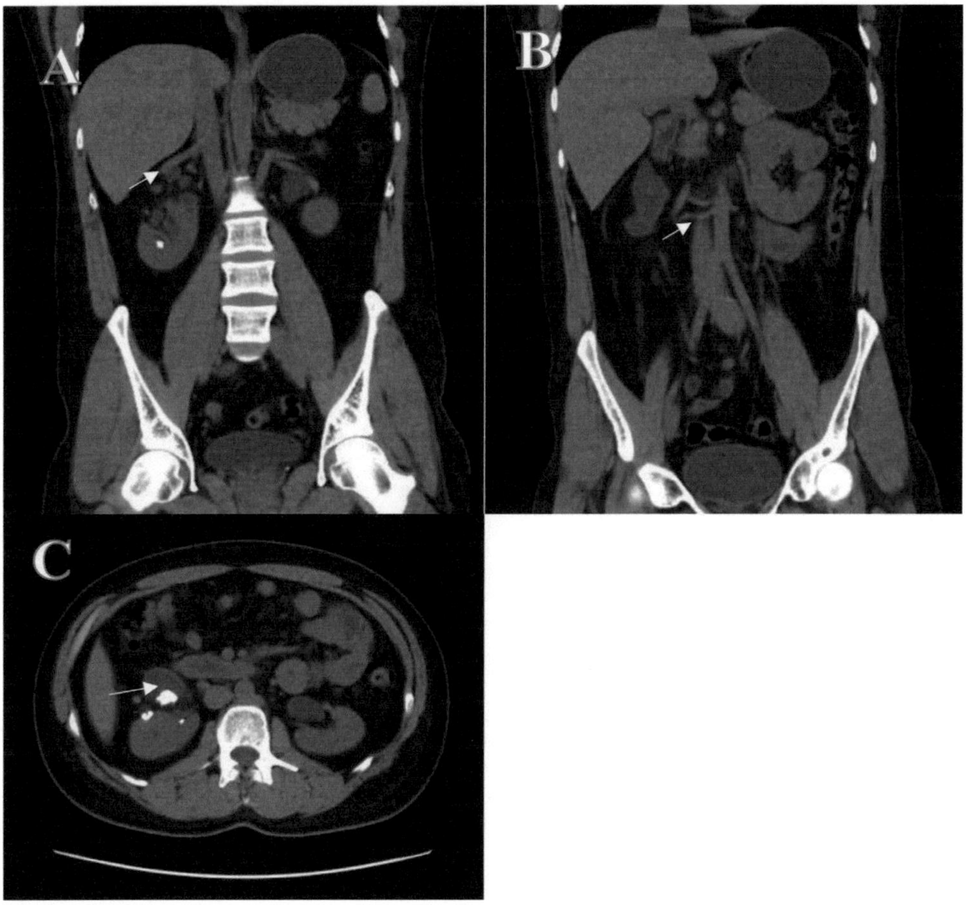

Figure 3.
A 29-year-old known case of urolithiasis, presented with acute colic imaging indicated 16 mm proximal ureteral stones and multiple small kidney stones (imaging not shown). Underwent RIRS and stenting. Stent removed after 2 months and was considered for ESWL for residual stones, however due to significant stone burden PCNL was advised. A renal vein (white arrow); B renal artery (white arrow) and C. malrotation and stones in renal pelvis and calyces.

5. Conclusions

Pregnancy is an independent risk factor for urolithiasis. In endemic areas, women with a history of urolithiasis, should undergo basic work to exclude kidney stones before planning pregnancy. Management of stones during pregnancy is complicated and compromised, particularly in the first and last trimester. Radiations should be avoided in the first trimester and interventions only when necessary.

Stones in urinary diversions are frequently seen. Stones can form as early as first year following diversion, so monitoring is important. Medical treatment is required after interventional treatment to avoid recurrence. Infection and obstruction are the two significant risk factors; infections are invariably present so perioperative antibiotics should be used. Most patients have hydronephrosis at presentation, so a PCN is always handy to have subsequent endourological interventions. CT is necessary to understand the anatomy, and loopogram is also helpful.

Stones in anomalous kidneys pose a challenging situation and require precise delineation of anatomy using a CT urogram. It helps to clarify calyceal and vascular anatomy. SWL is often not effective due to stone clearance issues [29]. PCNL and RIRS are the options of choice. RIRS is now considered the gold standard for most small-to-moderate size stone; ECIRS is an optional approach to malpositioned (ectopic) that often require laparoscopic guidance to PCNL; however, RIRS is a safer option.

Author details

Mohammad Hammad Ather
Aga Khan University, Pakistan

*Address all correspondence to: hammadather@gmail.com; hammd.ather@aku.edu

References

[1] Abufaraj M, Al Karmi J, Yang L. Prevalence and trends of urolithiasis among adults. Current Opinion in Urology. 2022;**32**(4):425-432

[2] Scales CD, Smith AC, Hanley JM, Saigal CS. Prevalence of kidney stones in the United States. European Urology. 2012;**62**:160-165

[3] Thongprayoon C, Vaughan LE, Chewcharat A, Kattah AG, Enders FT, Kumar R, et al. Risk of symptomatic kidney stones during and after pregnancy. American Journal of Kidney Diseases. 2021;**78**(3):409-417

[4] Spradling K, Zhang CA, Pao AC, Liao JC, Leppert JT, Elliott CS, et al. Risk of postpartum urinary stone disease in women with history of urinary stone disease during pregnancy. Journal of Endourology. 2022;**36**(1):138-142

[5] Somani BK, Dellis A, Liatsikos E, Skolarikos A. Review on diagnosis and management of urolithiasis in pregnancy: An ESUT practical guide for urologists. World Journal of Urology. 2017;**35**(11):1637-1649. DOI: 10.1007/s00345-017-2037-1 Epub 2017 Apr 19

[6] Ross AE, Handa S, Lingeman JE, Matlaga BR. Kidney stones during pregnancy: An investigation into stone composition. Urological Research. 2008;**36**(2):99-102

[7] White WM, Johnson EB, Zite NB, Beddies J, Krambeck AE, Hyams E, et al. Predictive value of current imaging modalities for the detection of urolithiasis during pregnancy: A multicenter, longitudinal study. The Journal of Urology. 2013;**189**(3):931-934. DOI: 10.1016/j.juro.2012.09.076 Epub 2012 Sep 24

[8] Shokeir AA, Mahran MR, Abdulmaaboud M. Renal colic in pregnant women: Role of renal resistive index. Urology. 2000;**55**(3):344-347. DOI: 10.1016/s0090-4295(99)00475-6

[9] Bold MS, Boyum JH, Potretzke AM, Rose CH, Atwell TD, Sviggum EB, et al. Journal of Ultrasound. 2021;**24**(4):397-402

[10] Lee JH, Roh HJ, Ahn JW, Kim JS, Choi JY, Lee SJ, et al. The diagnostic accuracy of magnetic resonance imaging for maternal acute adnexal torsion during pregnancy: Single-institution clinical performance review. Journal of Clinical Medicine. 2020;**9**(7):2209. DOI: 10.3390/jcm9072209

[11] Keenan RA, Hegarty NJ, Davis NF. Symptomatic Hydronephrosis and ureteral calculi in pregnancy: A narrative review with a proposed management protocol. Journal of Endourology. 2022;**36**(8):1099-1112. DOI: 10.1089/end.2021.0876

[12] Jung H, Osther PJ. Acute management of stones: When to treat or not to treat? World Journal of Urology. 2015;**33**(2):203-211. DOI: 10.1007/s00345-014-1353-y Epub 2014 Jul 2

[13] Theriault B, Morin F, Cloutier J. Safety and efficacy of Tamsulosin as medical expulsive therapy in pregnancy. World Journal of Urology. 2020;**38**(9):2301-2306. DOI: 10.1007/s00345-019-03022-z Epub 2019 Nov 25

[14] Elbatanouny AM, Ragheb AM, Abdelbary AM, Fathy H, Massoud AM, Abd El Latif A, et al. Percutaneous nephrostomy versus JJ ureteric stent as the initial drainage method in kidney stone patients presenting with acute

kidney injury: A prospective randomized study. International Journal of Urology. 2020;**27**(10):916-921

[15] Connelly ZM, Pilet H, Rees CD, McFerrin C, Azzawe A, Ahmed ME, et al. Do ureteral stent diameter and length or patient demographics play a role in stent encrustation? Canadian Urological Association Journal. 2022;**16**(9):E479-E483. DOI: 10.5489/cuaj.7815

[16] Asgari MA, Safarinejad MR, Hosseini SY, Dadkhah F. Extracorporeal shock wave lithotripsy of renal calculi during early pregnancy. BJU International. 1999;**84**(6):615-617

[17] Dai JC, Nicholson TM, Chang HC, Desai AC, Sweet RM, Harper JD, et al. Nephrolithiasis in pregnancy: Treating for two. Urology. 2021;**151**:44-53. DOI: 10.1016/j.urology.2020.06.097 Epub 2020 Aug 28

[18] Seth JH, Promponas J, Hadjipavlou M, Anjum F, Sriprasad S. Urolithiasis following urinary diversion. Urolithiasis. 2016;**44**(5):383-388

[19] van Hemelrijck M, Thorstenson A, Smith P, et al. Risk of in-hospital complications after radical cystectomy for urinary bladder carcinoma: Population-based follow-up study of 7608 patients. BJU International. 2013;**112**(8):1113-1120

[20] Ferriero M, Guaglianone S, Papalia R, et al. Risk assessment of stone formation in stapled orthotopic ileal neobladder. The Journal of Urology. 2015;**193**(3):891-896

[21] Hertzig LL, Iwaszko MR, Rangel LJ, Patterson DE, Gettman MT, Krambeck AE. Urolithiasis after ileal conduit urinary diversion: A comparison of minimally invasive therapies. The Journal of Urology. 2013;**189**(6): 2152-2157. DOI: 10.1016/j.juro.2012.12.003

[22] Turk TM, Koleski FC, Albala DM. Incidence of urolithiasis in cystectomy patients after intestinal conduit or continent urinary diversion. World Journal of Urology. 1999;**17**(5):305-307

[23] N'Dow J, Robson CN, Matthews JN, Neal DE, Pearson JP. Reducing mucus production after urinary reconstruction: A prospective randomized trial. The Journal of Urology. 2001;**165**(5):1433-1440

[24] Weizer AZ, Springhart WP, Ekeruo WO, Matlaga BR, Tan YH, Assimos DG, et al. Ureteroscopic management of renal calculi in anomalous kidneys. Urology. 2005;**65**(2):265-269

[25] Natsis K, Piagkou M, Skotsimara A, et al. Horseshoe kidney: A review of anatomy and pathology. Surgical and Radiologic Anatomy. 2014;**36**:517-526

[26] Hameed BM, Pietropaolo A, Naik N, Noronha C, JuliebøJones P, Mykoniatis I, et al. Role of three dimensional (3D) printing in endourology: An update from EAU young academic urologists (YAU) urolithiasis and endourology working group. Frontiers in Surgery. 2022;**9**:862348

[27] Lim EJ, Teoh JY, Fong KY, Emiliani E, Gadzhiev N, Gorelov D, et al. Propensity score-matched analysis comparing retrograde intrarenal surgery with percutaneous nephrolithotomy in anomalous kidneys. Minerva Urology and Nephrology. 2022;**74**:738-746

[28] Feng D, Zhang F, Liu S, Han P, Wei W. Efficacy and safety of the tranexamic acid in reducing blood loss and transfusion requirements during percutaneous nephrolithotomy: A

systematic review and meta-analysis of randomized controlled trials. Minerva Urologica e Nefrologica. 2020;**72**:579-585

[29] Tunc L, Tokgoz H, Tan MO, Kupeli B, Karaoglan U, Bozkirli I. Stones in anomalous kidneys: Results of treatment by shock wave lithotripsy in 150 patients. International Journal of Urology. 2004;**11**(10):831-836. DOI: 10.1111/j.1442-2042.2004.00916.x

Chapter 2

Renal Tract Stones – Diagnosis and Management

Ivan Thia and Matthew Chau

Abstract

This chapter explores the diagnosis as well as various methods for stone clearance and recent advancements in each of the avenues, so as to provide the avid reader an understanding of the basis of each intervention and new exciting technology that lay on the horizon. Each section is further subdivided such that it would be easy for readers to search and look up relevant information at a glance without having to read through the entirety of the chapter. Firstly, diagnosis of renal calculi is explored, as renal tract pain can mimic a variety of abdomino-pelvic conditions and cause the same constellation of symptoms. Evidence based investigation modalities are discussed. Subsequently, management of renal tract calculi are divided into conservative management with analgesia and medical expulsion therapy, extracorporeal shock wave lithotripsy, ureteropyeloscopy and laser lithotripsy, as well as percutaneous nephrolithotomy. The different stone size, composition, location and patient factors have all contributed to the different surgical options as detailed above. Each section end with a discussion of new and exciting innovations in each of the areas that may lead to even more efficient and safer interventions for the Urology of the future.

Keywords: urolithiasis, extracorporeal shockwave lithotripsy, Ureteropyeloscopy, percutaneous Nephrolithotomy, renal tract stones

1. Introduction

Renal tract calculi is a common presentation to an emergency department, and accounts for approximately 75% of presentations due to disorders of the genito-urinary system [1, 2]. One in ten people will have kidney stones in their lifetime. Recurrence of renal stones within five years approaches 50% [3]. However, not all renal tract calculi require surgical intervention, with 75–90% of these passing spontaneously with conservative management [3]. Despite this, the large volume of work in this area had prompted medical professionals, pharmaceutical companies and researchers alike to explore different avenues of approach to tackle this problem.

2. Diagnosis

2.1 History taking and examination

Haematuria is a common feature of ureteric calculi and is associated with approximately 82% of renal colic presentations [4]. Nausea and vomiting as well as lower urinary tract symptoms such as urinary urgency, frequency, dysuria or hesitancy are also often present. Associated fevers might be indicative of another inflammatory or infective processes or signal the presence of an infected obstructed kidney, which is a urological emergency.

A comprehensive examination of all abdominopelvic organ systems is essential to rule out other important or life-threatening conditions. It is important to remember that a diagnosis of renal colic does not exclude other concomitant medical conditions that may require more urgent attention.

2.2 Bedside tests

Patients who are thought to have renal stones should have the following tests: [5].

- urine dipstick analysis/urine culture
- full blood examination
- C-reactive protein
- serum urea, electrolyte, creatinine
- serum calcium and uric acid
- serum parathyroid hormone
- 24-hr urine metabolic screen

In conjunction with individual patient (eg age, comorbidities, renal function) and disease (stone, duration) factors, these investigations are important in helping to identify a subset of patients who are not suitable for conservative management, especially if there are markedly raised inflammatory markers or severe renal failure in the absence of other infections/inflammatory conditions.

2.3 Diagnostic imaging

Expedient imaging should not be delayed in patient populations suspected of suffering from renal tract calculi. Low-dose, non-contrast computed tomography (CT) of the kidneys, ureters and bladder (KUB) is the current gold-standard imaging of choice. CT KUB accurately determines stone location, size and density, aiding in surgical planning. Mimickers of renal colic such as appendicitis, cholecystitis, bowel obstruction, diverticulitis or adnexal pathology can also be reliably excluded. A meta-analysis by Worster et al. has demonstrated that CT KUB has a pooled sensitivity of 93.1% and specificity of 96.6% in detecting renal tract calculi [6]. Especially when patients are not obese with BMI <30 kg/m2, sensitivity for detection of stones >3 mm in size approaches 100% [7].

KUB ultrasonography (USS) is a useful alternative first-line imaging tool to pick up renal tract calculi, especially in patients who are more vulnerable to radiation exposure. USS KUB can also identify hydroureter and hydronephrosis secondary to post-renal obstruction. Unfortunately, sensitivity of USS is compromised due to its poor penetration of air, and is also highly dependent on factors such as operator skill and patient body habitus. Overall, KUB ultrasonography is safe, reproducible and inexpensive, with acceptable calculi detection rates for both renal (sensitivity 45%, specificity 88%) and ureteric (sensitivity 45%, specificity 94%) calculi [8].

X-Ray KUB readily picks up calcium containing calculi but are often inhibited by lack of sensitivity in picking up small renal tract calculi due to obscuring overlying bowel gas and presence of phleboliths. Brisbane et al. argues that XR KUB has value in monitoring of growth in cases of known renal calculi under surveillance and is less useful in the acute setting. This modality is not widely used anymore in tertiary centres to diagnose renal tract calculi where ultrasound and CT services are widely available.

3. Management of renal stones

The management of renal stones depend on many different factors and has to be individualised to patient needs and availability of resources. The table below lists some of the important factors to consider when determining the best therapeutic approach in a given scenario (**Table 1**).

There are various therapeutic options available to tackle renal and ureteral calculi, and one or more of these can be utilised in conjunction in the management of more complex cases. It is important to remember that not all calculi need surgical intervention, at least not at initial presentation, and that the above factors mentioned are dynamic and so should the therapeutic option selected.

The average diameter of a ureter measures 3-4 mm and a plethora of studies have been performed to determine factors that would predict spontaneous stone passage. The size of a stone is a known independent factor, with stone size <7 mm being the usual cutoff for trial of conservative management with analgesia. In a meta analysis by Pearce et al., likelihood of passage is 60% for stones smaller than 7 mm in a cohort of 1093 patients [9]. Another important factor studied was the location of the stone, with proximal ureteric stones generally having a lower spontaneous passage rate as compared to distal ureteric stones, although this finding was not universal. This is likely due to patients electing to undergo elective surgery for symptom control as well as lack of consistency in time period allowed for spontaneous passage before surgical intervention is organised. Medical expulsion therapy (MET) is frequently used in conjunction with analgesia to quicken passage of stone and reduce opioid use, thereby reducing risk of complications and providing symptomatic relief. Various medical therapies have been studied, and this will be discussed later in the chapter.

Extracorporeal shock wave lithotripsy (ESWL), first invented in 1980 in Germany, is still widely used to treat renal and ureteric calculi in healthy individuals with low stone burden. This approach to stone management is enticing as it allows for a minimally invasive method to fragment certain types of calculi in favourable locations, circumventing the need for more invasive options. ESWL is highly effective when applied to the appropriate patient population and should be incorporated into the repertoire of urological centres where available.

Factors Impacting Treatment of Renal Stones
Disease Factors: • Size • Location • Composition Patient Factors: • Renal anatomy - ptosis, horseshoe, pelvic, cross-fused, single functioning • Intrarenal anatomy - infundibulo-pelvic angle, infundibular length, infundibular width • Ureteric anatomy - strictures, pelvi-ureteric junction obstruction, duplication, ectopic • Medical comorbidities - including but not limited to coagulation status, pregnancy, cardiac/renal/respiratory function, immunosuppression, inflammatory or malignant conditions* • Surgical history - previous intervention for urological and non-urological pathologies, cardiothoracic and vascular procedures along retroperitoneum • Fitness for surgery • Superimposed infection • Preference • Compliance with follow up • Socioeconomic considerations - length of stay, morbidity, cost, legal • Geographic consideration - rural/urban/suburban Service Provision Factors: • Infrastructure/equipment availability • Technical expertise • Perioperative support availability • Imaging and radiology expertise availability

**Many medical factors are implicated in decision making, as they impact on the general fitness of an individual. The list stated is not exhaustive and a patient's comprehensive medical and medication history need to be taken into consideration when deciding on interventional therapies.*

Table 1.
Factors that impact the management of renal tract calculi.

Calculi fragmentation with laser lithotripsy is now the mainstay of nephrolithiasis management, and is widely employed for this purpose, with many urologists favouring its use due to its easy availability, flexibility, and ability to deal with almost any situation. Recent advancements in this field have allowed for greater and more accurate energy delivery, reduced retropulsion of stone fragments, and more customisable options to achieve better stone clearance with shorter operating times.

As for larger calculi >2 cm in size, percutaneous nephrolithotomy (PCNL) remains the gold standard surgical approach when attempting to achieve stone clearance. Patients do need to be counselled carefully as this procedure have higher preoperative complication rates as compared to the other interventions described. Open nephrolithotomy is now rarely used given its high morbidity rate and exclusive indications and is not within the scope of discussion in this chapter.

4. Conservative management

4.1 Analgesia

Non-obstructing renal calculi are generally asymptomatic and are frequently discovered incidentally in patients who have undergone either ultrasound or computed tomography (CT) imaging for other causes. The classic renal colic is triggered by an acute ureteric or calyceal obstruction leading to stretching of the corresponding proximal calyx, ureter, renal pelvis and/or peripelvic renal capsule [10, 11]. This pain cycle occurs in a predictable pattern and can be categorised into phases:

- acute - insidious, constant with intermittent exacerbation leading to severe pain, crescendo picture that lasts up to 6 hours
- constant - sustained, maximal pain intensity, lasts up to 4 hours
- relief - gradual diminishment of pain intensity, lasts up to 6 hours
- This cycle can and often does repeat till offending stone is removed or passed.

Renal colic is unique in its migratory nature and pattern of referred pain. Sensory innervation of the ureter is fed back via the sympathetic autonomic nervous system of levels T10-L2 [12]. Depending on the level of obstruction, the distribution of referred somatic pain varies. Intrarenal or proximal ureteric obstructing calculi tend to cause renal angle tenderness and flank pain. As the stone migrates into the middle and distal third of the ureter, patients with lower abdominal or groin pain that radiate to or from the scrotal/labial region [13]. Distal ureteric obstruction is also associated with storage lower urinary tract symptoms (LUTS) such as urinary urgency, frequency, dysuria and oliguria. However, it must be noted that renal colic is highly variable, and no one symptom or painful region can reliably predict the location of the offending stone.

4.2 Non-steroidal anti-inflammatory drugs (NSAIDs)

Renal colic is mediated by the secretion of prostaglandins secondary to local stimulation of the obstructing calculus. In turn, these prostagladins stimulate vasodilatation with greater permeability of glomerular afferent arterioles, increasing urine production and renal pelvic pressure in the acute phase [14]. The tight fibrous renal capsule does not allow room for expansion to accommodate this increased urine volume, with the increased intrarenal pressure manifesting as pain.

NSAIDs have been included in various guidelines and protocols across general practitioner and emergency department services as a first line analgesia drug for management of renal colic. Paracetamol and NSAIDs are non-selective or selective COX inhibitors and they inhibit the production of prostaglandins. Depending on formulation, this class of medication takes 3–7 days to reach maximal effect, causing a reduction in prostaglandin production, reducing glomerular filtration by up to 35%, thereby relieving renal pelvic pressure [15]. They also have local effects in reducing ureteric oedema and peristalsis, further reducing local stimulation of pain receptors [16–18]. This is evident with per-rectal (PR) administration of indomethacin for distal ureteric stones resulting in much better symptomatic pain relief as compared to other forms of analgesia.

Studies have shown that patients receiving NSAIDs as part of routine analgesia regimen for renal colic experience greater reduction in pain scores, require lower amounts of rescue analgesia for breakthrough pain and lower doses of opioids and therefore experience less opioid related side effects such as nausea and vomiting (5.8% vs. 19.5%) [19, 20]. Also, both oral PR NSAIDs reduce colic episodes when used as a regular medication, and reduce hospital admission rates by 28–57% [21]. However, it is worth noting that despite its benefits, NSAID administration does not reduce time to stone passage, nor does it increase the likelihood of spontaneous stone passage [22].

NSAIDs are versatile and come in different preparations including oral, intravenous, and PR formulations with analgesic effect seen from 30mins of administration. As only short courses of NSAIDs are required for symptomatic pain relief for renal colic, the potential side effects of exacerbating gastric irritation, renal and cardiac failure are rare even in patients with pre-existing disease if used with caution.

4.3 Opioids

Opioids are medications that work via binding to opioid receptors found predominantly in the nervous system and gastrointestinal tract, thereby producing its analgesic and anaesthetic effects [23]. There are many different opioids, binding to various receptors to varying degrees, either as agonists or antagonists, and these have found widespread application in the management of both acute and chronic pain. In the setting of renal colic, opioids mediate a quicker analgesic effect, although there is no significant difference found between opioid and NSAID for pain relief by 30mins. Also, opioids are ineffective in treating the underlying cause of renal colic, unlike NSAIDs, and require frequent, repeated dosing to achieve the desired pain relief, resulting in higher risk of gastrointestinal and neurodepression side effects.

4.4 Medical expulsive therapy (MET)

MET has been extensively studied as there is evidence that it reduces the time for passage of stones that would otherwise not have required surgical intervention, thereby achieving earlier symptomatic relief, reducing need for prolonged analgesia and risk of side effects, as well as reducing emergency department presentations and number of surgeries performed [24]. It was discovered that the distal ureters are rich with alpha-adrenergic receptors and that alpha blockers could possibly relax ureteral smooth muscle without impeding ureteral peristalsis as well as reduce ureteral oedema [25].

Alpha-blockers prove efficacious in increasing the rate of expulsion (RR 1.54, 95% CI: 1.29, 1.85; $p < 0.01$), reducing time to expulsion ($p < 0.01$), reducing analgesia use and providing relieve from renal colic ($p < 0.01$) [26]. The most well studied alpha-blocker is tamsulosin. The effect of this class of medication is most evident in larger stones (>5 mm) within the distal ureter. Newer, more selective medications of the same class such as silodosin (α1A) and naftopidil (α1D) show great promise, at the same time reducing the risk of experiencing the most common reported side effect of postural hypotension [27–30]. Alpha-blockers have also found a place as adjunct to surgical intervention, for example laser lithotripsy or external shockwave lithotripsy (ESWL), in aiding in the passage of residual stone fragments [31].

The use of calcium channel blockers, steroids and phosphodiesterase type 5 (PDE5) inhibitors are historic, and they have been shown to be inferior to alpha-blockers in several small studies. Therefore, the use of these medications should not be first line in MET.

4.5 Advancements

A multidisciplinary team approach to management of renal calculi has been shown to improve patient outcomes. The team should consist of a urologist, general practitioner, nurse practitioner. A radiologist, pharmacist and dietician should also be part of the team for the management and prevention of renal calculi. Conservative management of renal colic requires active monitoring, as stones that do not pass within 4 weeks require surgical removal to reduce risk of chronic renal scarring and atrophy.

5. Extracorporeal shockwave lithotripsy (ESWL)

ESWL was first invented in the 1970s and introduced as a novel method for management of renal tract stones in the 1980s, gaining widespread recognition and utility as a first-line treatment option [32]. Over the last 40 years, better technology and more advanced equipment have been developed, yet there has been little modification to the way the shock waves are generated or delivered to its intended target. The acoustic shockwave, a pressure pulse, produced by a lithotripter is responsible for both the fragmentation of renal tract calculi. Newer lithotripters have been built to focus on the efficient and safe delivery of these acoustic waves through body tissue to the intended target.

5.1 Basis of ESWL

A typical shockwave is short (~5 μs duration), with its energy spread over a large frequency range. Regardless of the type of lithotripter, the waveform of the shockwave produced is similar, consisting of a near instantaneous shock front, followed by a compressive phase, then a slowly diminishing tensile phase [33–35]. The difference in energy generated and magnitude of focal area determines the performance of the lithotripter.

An acoustic wave is created when an object moving through an air or fluid medium causes local compression and excitation of the medium surrounding it [36–38]. These molecules in turn excite their neighbours, leading to the successive propagation of the wave of energy. The speed at which the wave propagates depends on the medium in which it is travelling. When the object moves away from a medium, there is an opposite resultant disturbance called rarefaction, with its ensuing propagation leading to a tensile phase [39–41]. Shock waves generated by a lithotripter have compression and tensile phases travelling at different amplitude and speed, as the generation of a shockwave is nonlinear in nature [42–44].

The amount of energy delivered to the renal tract calculi is dependant on the wave intensity and its transmission or reflection. In relation to the above, acoustic impedance, the effective resistance of a medium to the propagation of an acoustic wave, is an important property [45–47]. The acoustic impedance of tissue, renal tract calculi, bone and air relative to water increases in orders of magnitude respectively, therefore it is important to minimise any air medium separating the lithotripter and the patient [48, 49]. As a comparison, up to 95% of energy would be transferred from water-to-stone via a shockwave, but only 0.1% of the same energy would be delivered water-to-air. Naturally, a flank approach through a predominantly tissue medium is favoured for an effective ESWL procedure.

Similar to the theory behind delivering radiotherapy, focusing and minimising diffraction of an energy source would ideally maximise damage to a particular area or object in question whilst minimising collateral injury as much as possible [50, 51]. Due to the nature of shockwave propagation, a focal area of high acoustic pressure is unavoidable. The size of the focal area is depending on how the lithotripter focuses the shockwave as well as the shape of the waveform it generates. A safe design feature would aim to deliver as large an acoustic pressure over as small a focal area as possible.

Shockwave generation can be created via a spark source (electrohydrolic lithotripter), magnetic repulsion (electromagnetic lithotripter) or crystal deformation (piezoelectric lithotripter) [52–55]. All of the above lithotripters would require a means of focusing shockwaves, whether it be an ellipsoid reflector, an acoustic lens or a spherical cap respectively. Once the shockwave is generated, coupling between the lithotripter and body is required for good transference of energy. Most modern lithotripters utilise an ellipsoid rubber couplant filled with water placed against a patient's body with a coupling gel in between to reduce any air pockets present, so as to deliver as much energy to the calculus as possible [56, 57].

5.2 Mechanism of action

The surface of a renal tract calculus is generally complex and irregular, meaning that the angle of incidence between a shockwave to stone is different at different regions. This results in a longitudinal compression wave as previously discussed, but also a perpendicular transverse shear wave that cause oscillation of molecules it passes through. These two waves travel at different speeds, reflect and refract again at different angles, and this interference causes high tensile stress within the calculus itself. Proposed mechanisms of stone fragmentation with ESWL include:

Spall fracture [58] - reflection of shockwave from posterior wall of calculus into incoming tensile phase pressure tail causes focal large tensile stress leading to material failure.

Shear stress [59] - interference between shear waves and compression waves exploit layered nature of calculus, leading to fracture along weakness of organic binding material between each layer of crystalline stone.

Superfocusing [60] - the amplification of stresses within a calculus due to its inherent geometry and elastic properties with initial shockwave reflected via diffraction and refraction to varying degrees.

Squeezing [60] - difference in property between calculus and surrounding urine/fluid medium results in circumferential hoop stress from shockwave travelling outside the calculus, leading to maximal axial tensile stress and material failure.

Cavitation [60] - collapsing bubbles predominantly on the proximal surface of the calculus created from the negative pressure tail of the acoustic pulse lead to generation of secondary shockwaves that are equally powerful.

Fatigue [60] - imperfections in stone material, coupled with repeated high stress insults lead to formation of cracks and eventual material breakdown.

5.3 Discussion

Due to the physical properties of wave formation and propagation, ESWL should be utilised selectively for management of renal calculi to achieve optimum success rates. Careful selection of patients should take into account of multiple factors, including:

- size of stone (renal calculi <20 mm, proximal or distal ureter calculi <10 mm)
- location (ureter, renal pelvis, renal calyx)
- stone composition
- patient habitus
- lithotripter availability

Snicorius et al. demonstrated that stone size or volume is the greatest prognostic factor in determining ESWL success, with an 80–85% stone clearance rate for stones <20 mm in size, down to 33–65% for stones >20 mm [61]. Stone clearance rates in the renal pelvis (86–89%), upper pole calyx (71–83%), inter polar calyx (73–84%) and lower pole calyx (37–68%) also differ significantly [61]. Stone composition determines material tensile and shear strength and therefore susceptibility to stress. For example, cystine and calcium oxalate monohydrate stones are difficult to comminute, and frequently fractures into larger fragments that are difficult to expulse, requiring further medical and surgical therapy [62]. Obesity translating into increased skin-to-stone distance is another independent predictive factor for stone failure [63]. Therefore, the importance of proper patient selection cannot be understated in improving treatment success rates.

Complications from ESWL is not uncommon and can result in devastating outcomes. As previously discussed, the mechanisms causing stone fragmentation also result in the same stress damage to body tissue. Due to the need to adjust the length of the focal area to penetrate deep into tissue onto stone, as well as patient movement or potential misalignment, many of the shockwaves pass directly onto surrounding tissue, which over prolonged and repeated insult will suffer collateral damage in spite of inherent tissue protective factors [64–66]. Mechanical stress from direct compression of tissue, variation in tissue impedance, expansion and collapsing cavitation bubbles all contribute to tissue damage [67]. Also, stone clearance may not be achieved satisfactorily, leading to secondary complications from residual stone fragments. Commonly cited complications and risk of individual events is described (**Table 2**).

ESWL complications	
Steinstrasse	4–7%
Renal colic	2–4%
Urinary tract infection	7–23%
Haematoma	4–19%
Cardiac dysrhythmia	11–59%
Bowel perforation, other solid organ haematoma	rare

Table 2.
ESWL complications and rates [68].

There is no general consensus regarding maximum number of shock waves that can be delivered per session, although small case series demonstrate >4000 shocks delivered, in an effort to reduce complication rates [69, 70]. Each session usually lasts 45-60mins, and repeated sessions can be performed to improve stone clearance rates. Insertion of a ureteric stent prior to commencement of ESWL therapy has not been shown to improve stone clearance. Another potential beneficial measure with weak evidence include commencing treatment at a low-power, low-frequency setting and subsequent stepwise power ramping may increase stone clearance rates and reduce tissue damage by inducing vasoconstriction and therefore renal bleeding [71–73].

Absolute contraindications of ESWL include: [74].

- pregnancy
- untreated urinary tract infection
- decompensated coagulopathy
- uncontrolled arrhythmia
- abdominal aortic aneurysm greater than 4 cm

5.4 Advancements

Greater understanding of shock wave generation and its mechanism of stone fragmentation have allowed for devices with producing waves with wider focal zones and lower peak pressures to reduce risk of injury yet at the same time improve stone fragmentation efficiency [75]. Secondly, experimental devices with twin sources firing in tandem or sequentially have been shown to improve stone fragmentation by increasing the number and amplitude of cavitation bubbles via a second pulse [76–78]. Combinations of piezoelectric with an electrohydraulic or piezoelectric with electromagnetic lithotripter have been experimented with.

Raskolnikov et al. describes a new ultrasound technique that takes this even further, with promising results in vitro. The new technology, utilising ultrasound technology and named burst wave lithotripsy (BWL), utilises a prolonged burst of consecutive, low amplitude ultrasound pulses rather than a single high amplitude shock wave produced in ESWL [79–81]. ESWL pulses lead to a focused fracture point, with resulting unsatisfactory stone fragmentation into large fragments that are then subsequently more difficult to break up with successive pulse waves. BWL, on the other hand, causes multiple fracture points to develop along the stone surface, with smaller fragments breaking off the main stone body, theoretically achieving better fragmentation. Fragment sizes are also more controlled depending on frequency of the ultrasound waves as compared to erratic fragment sizes produced by ESWL. Finally, BWL devices are more portable, less cumbersome and have the potential to be incorporated into pre-existing ultrasound devices, culminating in an exciting avenue of research for the future.

6. Ureteropyeloscopy with laser lithotripsy

Light amplification by stimulated emission of radiation, or laser for short, has found various applications in medicine since its inception in 1951, with dermatologist

Dr. Leon Goldman utilising a ruby laser to remove skin tattoos, while Dr. McGuff made use of one to ablate atherosclerotic plaques [82]. More recently, lasers are used extensively in the field of dentistry, cosmetic surgery, opthalmology, plastics surgery, and of course urology. In 1968, Mulvany first attempted to use a rubidium laser to fragment bladder stones, and has been a hallmark in the management of calculi in the urinary tract from the 80s [83].

6.1 Mechanism of action

All laser generators compose of an energy source, an active medium from which electromagnetic radiation is produced, and finally a resonant cavity with two mirrors (reflective and partially reflective) at each end [83]. The active semi-conductive, solid state medium (e.g Yttrium Aluminium Garnet, also known as YAG) is doped with excitable ions of neodynium, erbium, holmium or thulium [83]. An electric current is passed through the active medium, exciting atoms within its molecules, leading to the subsequent discharge of this energy as photons. Once the number of excited photons outnumbers the non-excited photons, a laser beam is produced. These laser beams have the same wavelength, travels in a single direction, and can be directed to travel in collimation with little divergence, with energy being delivered to a finite space with minimal dispersal [83]. Laser production is delivered in pulses, which can be controlled either with phase lock or a shutter mechanism, thereby reducing the potential for collateral tissue damage due to sustained exposure during procedures [83].

Laser-tissue interactions consist of photomechanical and photothermal processes [82]. Photomechanical processes induced by laser directed at calculi is akin to the mechanisms discussed for ESWL in previous sections. The deposition of energy from the laser beam around a calculi causes a transient, unstable stress wave leading to spallation or mechanical disruption, as well as formation and collapse of cavitation bubbles, both of which cause stress fractures to occur along the stone matrix and the ejection of ablated material through recoil [82]. Photothermal processes are a result of direct absorption of energy by the calculi and depending on the temperature induced, results in ablation, fragmentation and eventual vaporisation of material [82]. This energy transfer occurs via direct photon absorption by the calculi or indirect transfer from surrounding water through explosive vaporisation [82].

6.2 Laser fibre construct

There are certain requirements to be met for a laser fibre to be able to deliver photons from its energy source to its intended target: [84–86].

- light travelling without impediment
- minimal energy loss or dissipation
- low back-burn
- easy insertion and travel within ureteroscopes (semi-rigid and flexible) or nephroscopes
- lightweight with ease of transport and storage

- able to sustain prolonged use
- flexible, able to bend and maintain use

To that end, a laser fibre is usually constructed from a fused silica-glass compound at its core, with multiple layers of cladding around it to reduce risk of fibre failure due to bending and heat absorption [87].

Fibre tip design is vital in determining ease of use of the fibre as well as minimising back-burning, whereby the tip of the fibre with its covering jacket might be damaged due to overheating or contact with calculi [88]. A variety of tips are in use today, namely the flat tip and the ball tip. Other advancements including usage of a hollow steel tip (increased durability), tapered fibre (increased flexibility) and inverse tapered fibre (reduced overheating) have also been experimented with success [88].

6.3 Laser parameters

As discussed, photothermal processes induce dehydration, vaporisation and carbonisation of the stone surface when a critical thermal threshold is reached, and is effective in all stone types [89, 90]. As this process is going on, the photomechanical processes then exploit this weakness, leading to material failure, fragmentation, and retropulsion through cavitation bubble disruption. Ease of calculus fragmentation is dependent on both stone and laser properties. There are multiple parameters that determine or influence the laser beam, with the following three described being the most commonly calibrated by urologists during a procedure: [91].

- frequency: number of pulses emitted per second (Hz)
- pulse energy: total energy power of the laser pulse (J)
- pulse duration: time during which the laser pulse energy remains above half its maximum value

Generally, to fragment and basket a calculus in the ureter, typical settings used would be one of high pulse energy and low frequency [92]. To dust a stone, on the contrary, a low pulse energy and high frequency is employed [92]. Pulse duration is another important parameter gaining more scrutiny as it influences efficiency of calculus fragmentation. Long-pulse mode reduces stone fibre back-burn without sacrificing stone retropulsion. Newer energy sources allow for the Moses effect, whereby a shorter, lower energy pulse is first projected to create a cavitation bubble followed by a longer, higher energy pulse which improves fragmentation efficiency [93–95].

Also it must be noted that increasing fibre size does not correlate with increased energy delivery. Conversely, larger fibre sizes are associated with increased energy dispersion and poorer fragmentation rates [96].

6.4 Dusting versus fragmentation

Dusting of calculi refer to the use of low energy, high frequency laser pulses to break them down to dust or minute fragments, after which the larger residual fragments can be broken down further with the "whirlpool" and "popcorning" method [97]. The fragmentation technique aims to break down calculi into larger, bite-sized fragments measuring ~3 mm or so and retrieving them with a basket, thereby leaving the patient stone free [98]. Both methods are widely used, and although Chatloff et al. demonstrated that re-presentations to the emergency department was more frequent with the dusting group (30–3%), Humphreys et al. found no difference in re-presentations or complication rates between the two groups, with the fragmentation group requiring a longer operative time [98, 99].

The method of choice should depend on the stone composition, size, location and patient preference. Dusting would arguably reduce the need for use of a ureteric access sheath and stent, with a shorter operating time whilst increasing risk of subsequent renal colic. Fragmentation, on the other hand, necessitates the use of a ureteric access sheath with increased risk of ureteric trauma, as well as requiring stent placement post-operatively.

6.5 Safety and complications

Safety principles when operating laser equipment include: [100].

deploying laser fibre at a safe distance away from the tip of ureteroscope and not close to or within it

- directing laser fibre tip away from tissue surfaces
- maintaining irrigation throughout procedure
- minimise prolonged, continuous laser activation
- Injury to human tissue could be due to direct contact or indirect thermal damage. Complications from laser lithotripsy are rare, but can include operator eye injuries, ureteral injuries/perforations, bladder injuries/perforations, air emboli, bleeding and skin burns [100].

6.6 Future directions

The Holmium:YAG laser has been the dominant system utilised globally over the last 20 years, with the newer Thulium fibre laser (TFL) system showing major improvements over its predecessor. Apart from offering the most comprehensive modifiable laser parameters to improve stone ablation efficiency, it also has greater water absorption peak, meaning risk of optical or tissue damage is reduced to a quarter as compared to the Holmium:YAG system [101]. The TFL also uses nine times less energy, is more flexible and breaks calculi into smaller fragment by virtue of its smaller fibre. It also boasts a more manoeuvrable energy system that is seven times smaller and eight times lighter than a conventional Holmium:YAG model [102, 103]. Future improvements with the TFL include being able to use different endoscopic instruments simultaneously as well as miniaturisation of instruments with important applications.

6.7 Conclusion

Laser lithotripsy is an extremely flexible procedure that could be used in most situations to break up stones of any composition. Indeed, it is the most widely used technique for stone fragmentation at present, quickly overtaking ESWL and percutaneous nephrolithotomy (PCNL) with most guidelines recommending it as first-line therapy in various situations.

The only absolute contraindication to the use of laser lithotripsy is untreated urinary tract infections that may lead to severe urosepsis.

7. Percutaneous nephrolithotomy (PCNL)

7.1 Introduction

PCNL is a minimally-invasive surgical technique that allows removal of stones through a percutaneous access, typically through the back and into the kidney. The first nephroscopy was described by Rupel and Brown in 1941 in which a rigid cystoscope was passed into the kidney during open surgery [104]. Shortly after, Goodwin placed the first nephrostomy tube after performing the first antegrade nephrostogram. This lead to Fernström and Johansson to describe the first technique of stone extraction through percutaneous access under radiological guidance in 1976. With ongoing advancement of technology starting from the Godfathers of endourology such as Kurt Amplatz and Arthur Smith, the PCNL technique has developed into a reliable and effective technique for stone extraction.

PCNL monotherapy, or in combination with ESWL, is currently the most effective treatment option for patients with large stone burden. Stone free rate is seen up to 80–90% after PCNL for renal calculi and 86% for proximal ureteric stones. Multiple tracts allow for the successful treatment with a single surgical session in almost all stone burden.

PCNL is reserved for patients with large stone burden in the kidney and upper ureter, as seen in patients with complete or partial staghorn calculi, renal stones larger than 2 cm, proximal ureteric stones larger than 1 cm and multiple stones between 1 and 2 cm [105–107]. Patients with large (>1 cm) lower pole stones where retrograde access is difficult, may also benefit from PCNL. Additionally, patients who have failed conservative options such as retrograde lithotripsy or shockwave lithotripsy may also be considered for PCNL. Given the more invasive nature of PCNL, patients with uncorrected coagulopathies are excluded from PCNL due to the high risk of bleeding. Untreated urinary tract infections are another absolute contraindication for performing PCNL. Careful consideration should be made for patients with single kidneys.

Pre-operative assessment of patient prior to PCNL should include a complete medical history and physical examination. Assessment of the before mentioned contraindications should be addressed. Antiplatelet and anticoagulation therapy should be assessed and individualised to each patient in order to balance the bleeding risk with the thromboembolic risk. The underlying pathology for each patient necessitating anticoagulation/antiplatelet therapy differs and should be taken into account when deciding on the cessation period and reinitiating timing [108–110]. Bridging therapy may be required in patients with high thromboembolic risks such as mechanical prosthetic heart valves. If medically suitable, antiplatelet and anticoagulation therapy should be withheld according to local protocols. Current literature recommends cessation of antiplatelet therapy 7 days prior to surgery. Anticoagulation therapy cessation depends on the type of therapy and patient ability to excrete medication. Preoperative urine culture should be performed to exclude UTI and appropriate antibiotic therapy given. Broad-spectrum antibiotics can also be given prophylactic to assist with the bacteria colonised on calculi [105]. Anaesthesia review should also be obtained.

Preoperative planning with computed tomography (CT) scans is essential for planning of percutaneous access. CT allows identification of stone burden, location and puncture trajectory. The kidney typically lies within the retroperitoneum on the psoas and quadratus lumborum muscles. Significant structures surround the kidney includes the ribs, liver, duodenum and colon on the right, and the ribs, pancreas (tail), spleen and colon on the left. Bilaterally, the diaphragm and pleura lie in close relation with the upper pole of the kidney. Planning of puncture site and trajectory should consider these surrounding structures as well assessment of complex anatomy such as hepatomegaly or retrorenal colon. It is also particularly useful in cases of anatomical variations such as horseshoe kidneys, congenital renal anomalies, transplanted kidney, morbid obesity and evaluation of adjacent visceral structures [105].

7.2 Approaches

Patients are typically positioned in prone, prone-flexed, supine, supine oblique or split-leg modified lateral positions. The ideal position for optimal access is still controversial and is usually determined in a case-by-case method. Complex anatomy, patient characteristics (such as body habitus) and surgeon training are all factors to be considered.

PCNL is performed with percutaneous access into the renal collecting system. There are multiple modalities of imaging that can be used to assist with access. Common modalities include fluoroscopy, ultrasound, CT or MRI guidance and endoscopic guidance. Often, the surgeon urologist prefers to obtain their own access over interventional radiology as it allows targeting of calyces that maximise calculi access.

Most urologists are familiar with fluoroscopy guided percutaneous access, clarity of visibility of their needle and guide wire and the ability to visualise the calculi [111, 112]. During fluoroscopic puncture of the calyx, radiation exposure should be considered as the fluoroscopic screening time during PCNL is higher than most other urological procedures. At the beginning of a procedure, cystoscopy and retrograde placement of a ureteral catheter or access sheath assists with injection on contrast. The renal collecting system is initially opacified with contrast to assist with localising the target calyx.

Ultrasonographic guidance uses real-time diagnostic ultrasonography (US) to identify a renal collecting system to target calyces. Agarwal et al. have identified the overall success rate of this technique to be 88–99%. US utilises no radiation, minimising the radiation exposure for patients and staff, making it safe for pregnant and paediatric patients. USS allows visualisation of soft tissues including surrounding structures, which assists with avoiding iatrogenic injury to the surrounding structures. US can be more difficult in patients without a dilated system, as visualisation of the calyces will be more difficult. Instruments such as wires and needles are harder to identify on US.

Once access into the collecting system is gained, a nephroscope is introduced to identify the stone. Stone extraction can be performed by different methods.

7.2.1 Manual

If calculi are smaller than 1 cm in size, they may be manually extracted through the access sheath with a grasper. Graspers can be toothed or non-toothed. Other devices such as stone baskets, made of soft, pliable material, can be used as well.

7.2.2 Laser lithotripsy

As previously described, laser can be used to fragment stones for extraction.

7.2.3 Ultrasonic lithotripsy

The use of ultrasonic lithotripter is the author's preferred method of stone extraction. The setup typically includes a handheld device, a metal rod containing the working channel and master control unit [112–114]. A handheld device is used to convert electrical current into vibration waves by utilising a piezoelectric crystal. The ultrasonic waves are translated down a metal rod, which fragments the stone when brought into direct contact. Variable suction is also applied through the working channel to allow stone removal, post-fragmentation. Heat energy is produced as a byproduct though, a risk of thermal injury to both the patient and surgeon needs to be considered when being used. Current technology combines the use of ultrasonic energy with ballistic energy to increase the rate of stone clearance. Ballistic devices repeatedly drive a solid probe into the target to drill and fragment stones. Similar to a jackhammer, it is particularly useful in hard stones resistant to ultrasonic lithotripsy. The lack of heat production and dissipation mitigates the thermal injury risk that is associated with ultrasonic lithotripsy.

Calyceal stone clearance is confirmed with a combination of careful inspection of the collecting system and ensuring all shadows on fluoroscopy have been removed. Following completion of lithotripsy, depending on surgeon preference, a ureteral stent, nephrostomy tubes or nothing may be inserted. Nephrostomy tube, usually a foley catheter, insertion may assist with a second access (relook PCNL or emergency access) and provide low intrarenal pressure to assist with haemostasis. Ureteral stents may assist with residual stone fragments or dust passage. In very select patients who are deemed to have total clearance and without pelvi-ureteric junction oedema, stent and nephrostomy tubes may be omitted.

7.2.4 Endoscopic combined intrarenal surgery (ECIRS)

In recent years, the popularisation of ECIRS has been experienced with studies supporting the efficacy and efficiency of stone clearance during PCNL. Initially described in 2008 by Scoffone et al., it describes a technique that combines retrograde and antegrade access to large and complex renal stones using both rigid and flexible endoscopes [115]. Cracco et al. published a systematic review in 2020 that updated the results and outcomes of ECIRS since its popularisation [116]. Studies have shown ECIRS demonstrates better stone clearance rates in a single surgical procedure (61–97% with ECIRS vs. 57–78% with standard PCNL) with reduced number of percutaneous punctures. ECIRS has reported similar complications rates when compared to standard PCNL techniques, with the majority of complications reported being low grade. However, ECIRS is associated with lower risk of bleeding complications, which is likely related to the single puncture site compared to multiple punctures by standard techniques. The reduced need for multiple access is an important factor that reduces the adherent risk of haemorrhage, infection and operative time.

7.3 Complications

Common complications from PCNL include mild bleeding immediately post-operative, residual stone burden requiring a second operation, recurrent (new) stone

PCNL complications	
Haematuria	4–7%
Haemorrhage	
Requiring Transfusion	0.6–11.2%
Requiring Intervention	0.3–2.0%
Fever	11–32%
Sepsis	0.8–1.8%
Recurrent stone formation	50%
Residual stone requiring another surgery	4.8–20%
Bowel or surrounding organ injury	0.3–2%

Table 3.
PCNL complications [118].

formation and urinary tract infections [105, 117]. Less common complications include haemorrhage, sepsis requiring intensive care admission, pneumothorax/hydrothorax. Moderately severe bleeding from the kidney or pseudoaneurysms requiring interventional radiological intervention for embolisation, failure of access to the kidney, infection of the nephrostomy puncture site and anaesthetic or cardiovascular related complications. Extremely rare, major damage to major renal vessels may result in emergency nephrectomy to control bleeding. Urine leak, bowel, spleen or liver injury is rare, but may also occur. Complications are outlined in **Table 3**. Both clinical and biochemical assessment is required in order to identify complications early for management.

During a PCNL, haemorrhagic complications may occur from the puncture, tract dilatation and stone fragmentation, thus careful pre-operative planning is required to prevent these from occurring. Lee et al. described body mass index (BMI) as a contributing factor to bleeding in PCNL [110]. Conversely, Said et al. and Gok et al. found no significant correlation with this [108, 119]. Yesil et al. had identified previous open abdominal surgery, stone treatment (ESWL) and those with previous PCNL all held a higher risk of haemorrhagic complications [120]. This was backed by Said et al. and Arora et al. A more significant risk factor for haemorrhagic complications is diabetes mellitus. It has been hypothesised that the arteriosclerosis can be the source of bleeding post-PCNL in diabetic patients. The other identified risk factor is the presence of pre-operative urinary tract infections. An urinary tract infection can cause inflammation of renal parenchyma that makes it more friable and impairs coagulation, which results in haemorrhagic complications. Interestingly, current literature shows no convincing evidence of correlation between bleeding post PCNL with age, stone position and anticoagulation use [108, 109, 119, 121]. Despite no correlation, the authors still recommend careful pre-operative planning with anticoagulants and anti-platelet therapy cessation.

8. Summary

There are many approaches to managing renal and ureteric stones as mentioned, and careful patient selection is required for optimal outcomes. **Tables 4** and **5** detail current guideline recommendations regarding treatment modality of choice listed by

Renal calculus	
Larger than 20 mm	1. PCNL 2. URS or ESWL
10-20 mm	1. URS or ESWL 2. PCNL
Lower pole 10-20 mm (unfavourable)	1. URS 2. PCNL 3. ESWL
Lower pole 10-20 mm (favourable)	1. URS or ESWL 2. PCNL
Smaller than 10 mm	1. URS or ESWL

Table 4.
Current guideline recommendations for the management of renal calculi.

Proximal ureteric calculi	
Larger than 10 mm	1. URS or ESWL
Smaller than 10 mm	1. ESWL 2. URS
Distal ureteric calculi	
Larger than 10 mm	1. URS 2. ESWL
Smaller than 10 mm	1. URS or ESWL

Table 5.
Current guideline recommendations for management of ureteric calculi.

the European Association of Urology according to stone size and location. These are meant to help guide clinician decision making, bearing in mind each patients' individual unique circumstance and requirements.

Author details

Ivan Thia* and Matthew Chau
Fiona Stanley Hospital, Western Australia, Australia

*Address all correspondence to: ivan.thia@health.wa.gov.au

References

[1] Thia I, Saluja M. An update on the Management of Renal Colic. AJGP. 2021;**50**(7):445-449. DOI: 10.31128/AJGP-11-20-5751

[2] Australian Institute of Health and Welfare. Media Release: Emergency Department Care. Bruce, ACT: AIHW, 2020. Available at www.aihw.gov.au/reports-data/myhospitals/sectors/emergency-department-care [Accessed 23 July 2022].

[3] Pathan SA, Mitra B, Bhutta ZA, et al. A comparative, epidemiological study of acute renal colic presentations to emergency departments in Doha, Qatar, and Melbourne, Australia. International Journal of Emergency Medicine. 2018;**11**(1):1. DOI: 10.1186/s12245-017-0160-9

[4] Mefford JM, Tungate RM, Amini L, et al. A comparison of urolithiasis in the presence and absence of microscopic haematuria in the emergency department. The Western Journal of Emergency Medicine. 2017;**18**(4):775-779. DOI: 10.5811/westjem.2017.4.33018

[5] Jindai G, Ramachandani P. Acute flank pain secondary to urolithasis: Radiologic evaluation and alternate diagnoses. Radiologic Clinics of North America. 2007;**45**(3):395-410, vii. DOI: 10.1016/j.rcl.2007.04.001

[6] Worster A, Preya I, Weaver B, Haines T. The accuracy of noncontrast helical computed tomogaphy versus intravenous pyelography in the diagnosis of suspected acute urolithiasis: A meta-analysis. Annals of Emergency Medicine. 2002;**40**(3):280-286. DOI: 10.1067/mem.2002.126170

[7] Zheng X, Liu Y, Li M, Wang Q, Song B. Dual-energy computed tomography for characterizing urinary calcified calculi and uric acid calculi: A meta-analysis. European Journal of Radiology. 2016;**85**(10):1843-1848. DOI: 10.1016/j.ejrad.2016.08.013

[8] Smith-Bindman R, Aubin C, Bailitz J, et al. Ultrasonography versus computed tomography for suspected nephrolithiasis. The New England Journal of Medicine. 2014;**371**(12):1100-1110. DOI: 10.1056/NEJMoa1404446

[9] Pearce E, Clement KD, Yallappa S, Aboumarzouk OM. Likelihood of distal ureteric calculi to pass spontaneously: Systematic review and cumulative analysis of the placebo arm of randomised-controlled trials. Urologia Internationalis. 2021;**105**(1-2):71-76 Available from Pubmed

[10] Dewar MJ, Chin JL. Chronic renal pain: An approach to investigation and management. Canadian Urological Association Journal. 2018;**12**(6Suppl 3):S167-SS70. DOI: 10.5489/cuaj.5327

[11] Portis AJ, Sundaram CP. Diagnosis and initial management of kidney stones. American Family Physician. 2001;**63**(7):1329-1339

[12] Bueschen AJ. Flank pain. In: Walker HK, Hall WD, Hurst JW, editors. Clinical Methods: The History, Physical, and Laboratory Examinations. 3rd ed. Boston, MA: Butterworths; 1990. pp. 845-846

[13] Menon M, Parulkar BG, Drach GW. Urinary lithiasis: Etiology, diagnosis and medical management. In: Walsh PC, Retik AB, Vaughan ED Jr, Wein AJ, editors. Campbell's Urology. 7th ed. Philadelphia, PA: WB Saunders; 1998. pp. 2661-2733

[14] Shokeir AA. Renal colic: Pathophysiology, diagnosis and treatment. European Urology. 2001;**39**(3):241-249. DOI: 10.1159/000052446

[15] Davenport K, Waine E. The role of non-steroidal anti-inflammatory drugs in renal colic. Pharmaceuticals (Basel). 2010;**3**(5):1304-1310. DOI: 10.3390/ph3051304

[16] Pathan SA, Mitra B, Straney LD, et al. Delivering safe and effective analgesia for management of renal colic in the emergency department: A double-blind multigroup, randomised controlled trial. Lancet. 2016;**387**(10032):1999-2007. DOI: 10.1016/S0140-6736(16)00652-8

[17] Pathan SA, Mitra B, Cameron PA. A systematic review and meta-analysis comparing the efficacy of nonsteroidal anti-inflammatory drugs, opioids, and paracetamol in the treatment of acute renal colic. European Urology. 2018;**73**(4):583-595. DOI: 10.1016/j.eururo.2017.11.001

[18] Cole RS, Fry CH, Shuttleworth KE. The action of the prostaglandins on isolated human ureteric smooth muscle. British Journal of Urology. 1988;**61**(1):19-26. DOI: 10.1111/j.1464-410x.1988.tb09155.x

[19] Perlmutter A, Miller L, Trimble LA, Marion DN, Vaughan ED Jr, Felsen D. Toradol, an NSAID used for renal colic, decreases renal perfusion and ureteral pressure in a canine model of unilateral ureteral obstruction. The Journal of Urology. 1993;**149**(4):926-930. DOI: 10.1016/s0022-5347(17)36261-4

[20] Sivrikaya A, Celik OF, Sivrikaya N, Ozgur GK. The effect of diclofenac sodium and papaverine on isolated human ureteric smooth muscle. International Urology and Nephrology. 2003;**35**:479-483. DOI: 10.1023/b:urol.0000025618.68752.5b

[21] Schjerning Olsen AM, Fosbøl EL, Lindhardsen J, et al. Duration of treatment with nonsteroidal anti-inflammatory drugs and impact on risk of death and recurrent myocardial infarction in patients with prior myocardial infarction: A nationwide cohort study. Circulation. 2011;**123**(20):2226-2235. DOI: 10.1161/CIRCULATIONAHA.110.004671

[22] Golzari SE, Soleiman H, Rahmani F, Mehr NZ, et al. Therapeutic approaches for renal colic in the emergency department: A review article. Anesth. Pain Medicine. 2014;**4**(1):e16222 Available from: Pubmed

[23] Holdgate A, Pollack T. Systematic review of the relative efficacy of non-steroidal anti-inflammatory drugs and opioids in the treatment of acute renal colic. BMJ. 2004;**328**(7453):1401 Available from: Pubmed

[24] Dellabella M, Milanese G, Muzzonigro G. Randomized trial of the efficacy of tamsulosin, nifeipine and phloroglucinol in medical expulsive therapy for distal ureteral calculi. The Journal of Urology. 2005;**174**(1):167-172. DOI: 10.1097/01.ju.0000161600.54732.86

[25] Wang H, Man LB, Huang GL, Li GZ, Wang JW. Comparative efficacy of tamsulosin versus nifedipine for distal ureteral calculi: A meta-analysis. Drug Design, Development and Therapy. 2016;**10**:1257-1265. DOI: 10.2147/DDDT.S99330

[26] Wood KD, Gorbachinsky I, Gutierrez J. Medical expulsive therapy. Indian Journal of Urology. 2014;**30**(1):60-64. DOI: 10.4103/0970-1591.124209

[27] Oestreich MC, Vernooij RW, Sathianathen NJ, et al. Alpha-blockers after shock wave lithotripsy for renal or ureteral stones in adults.

Cochrane Database of Systematic Reviews. 2020;**11**:CD013393. DOI: 10.1002/14651858.CD013393.pub2

[28] Ding H, Ning Z, Dai Y, Shang P, Yang L. The role of silodosin as a new medical expulsive therapy for ureteral stones: A meta-analysis. Renal Failure. 2016;**38**(9):1311-1319. DOI: 10.1080/0886022X.2016.1215221

[29] Pickard R, Starr K, MacLennan G, et al. Medical expulsive therapy in adults with ureteric colic: A multicentre, randomised, placebo-controlled trial. Lancet. 2015;**386**(9991):341-349. DOI: 10.1016/S0140-6736(15)60933-3

[30] Ye Z, Zeng G, Yang H, et al. Efficacy and safety of tamsulosin in medical expulsive therapy for distal ureteral stones with renal colic: A multicenter, randomized, double-blinded, placebo-controlled trial. European Urology. 2018;**73**(3):385-391. DOI: 10.1016/j.eururo.2017.10.033

[31] Hollingsworth J, Canales BK, Rogers MA, et al. Alpha blockers for treatment of ureteric stones: Systematic review and meta-analysis. BMJ. 2016;**355**:i6112. DOI: 10.1136/bmj.i6112

[32] Wess O, Talatti JJ, et al. Physics and Technique of Shock Wave Lithotripsy. Urolithiasis. London: Springer-Verlag; 2012. pp. 301-311. Available from:. DOI: 10.1007/978-1-4471-4387-1_38

[33] Holmes S, Whitfield HN. The current status of lithotripsy. British Journal of Urology. 1991;**68**:337-344

[34] Kerbl K, Rehman J, Landman J, et al. Current management of urolithiasis: Progress or regress? Journal of Endourology. 2002;**16**:281-288

[35] Lingeman JE, Newmark J. Adverse bioeffects of shock-wave lithotripsy. In: Coe FL et al., editors. Kidney Stones: Medical and Surgical Management. Philadelphia: Lippincott Raven; 1996. pp. 605-614

[36] Evan AP, Willis LR, Lingeman JE, McAteer JA. Renal trauma and the risk of long-term complications in shock wave lithotripsy. Nephron. 1998;**78**:1-8

[37] Ueda S, Matsuko K, Yamashita T, et al. Perirenal hematoma caused by SWL with EDAP LT-01 lithotriptor. Journal of Endourology. 1993;**7**:11-15

[38] IEC61846. Ultrasonics – pressure pulse lithotripters – characteristics of fields. Ultrasonics T, editor. 1998

[39] Dreyer T, Riedlinger RE, Steiger E. Experiments on the relation of shock wave parameters to stone disintegration. In: 16th International Congress on Acoustics. Seattle, WA, USA: Acoustical Society of America; 1998

[40] Fry FJ, Dins KA, Reilly CR, Goss SA. Losses in tissue associated with finite amplitude ultrasound transmission. Ultrasound in Medicine & Biology. 1989;**15**:481-497

[41] Hynynen K. The role of nonlinear ultrasound propagation during hyperthermia treatments. Medical Physics. 1991;**18**:1156-1163

[42] Hynynen K. Review of ultrasound therapy. In: IEEE Ultrasonics Symposium Proceedings: An International Symposium; 1997; Toronto, Canada. New York: IEEE; 1997

[43] Bailey MR, Khokhlova VA, Sapozhnikov OA, et al. Physical mechanisms of the therapeutic effect of ultrasound (a review). Acoustical Physics. 2003;**49**:369-388

[44] Coleman AJ, Saunders JE, Preston RC, Bacon DR. Pressure

waveforms generated by a Dornier extracorporeal shockwave lithotriptor. Ultrasound in Medicine & Biology. 1987;**13**:651-657

[45] 26.Coleman AJ, Saunders JE, Crum LA, Dyson M. Acoustic cavitation generated by an extracorporeal shockwave lithotriptor. Ultrasound in Medicine & Biology. 1987;**13**:69-76

[46] Crum LA. Cavitation microjets as a contributory mechanism for renal calculi disintegration in ESWL. The Journal of Urology. 1988;**140**:1587-1590

[47] Atchley AA, Prosperetti A. The crevice model of bubble nucleation. The Journal of the Acoustical Society of America. 1989;**86**(3):1065-1084

[48] Philipp A, Delius M, Scheffczyk C, et al. Interaction of lithotriptor-generated shock waves with air bubbles. The Journal of the Acoustical Society of America. 1993;**93**:2496-2509

[49] Sass W, Matura E, Dreyer HP, et al. Lithotripsy-mechanisms of the fragmentation process with focussed shock waves. Electromedica. 1993;**61**:2-12

[50] Zhong P, Cioanta I, Cocks FH, Preminger GM. Inertial cavitation and associated acoustic emission produced during electrohydraulic shock wave lithotripsy. The Journal of the Acoustical Society of America. 1997;**101**:2940-2950

[51] Pishchalnikov YA, Sapozhnikov OA, Bailey MR, et al. Cavitation bubble cluster activity in the breakage of kidney stones by lithotriptor shockwaves. Journal of Endourology. 2003;**17**:435-446

[52] Paterson RF, Lifshitz DA, Lingeman JE, et al. Stone fragmentation during shock wave lithotripsy is improved by slowing the shock wave rate: Studies with a new animal model. The Journal of Urology. 2002;**168**:2211-2215

[53] Agarwal R, Singh VR. A comparative study of fracture strength, ultrasonic properties and chemical constituents of kidney stones. Ultrasonics. 1991;**29**:89-90

[54] Zhong P, Preminger GM. Mechanisms of differing stone fragility in extracorporeal shockwave lithotripsy. Journal of Endourology. 1994;**8**:263-268

[55] Chaussy C, Brendel W, Schmiedt E. Extracorporeally induced destruction of kidney stones by shock waves. Lancet. 1980;**2**:1265-1268

[56] Chaussy C. Extracorporeal Shock Wave Lithotripsy: New Aspects in the Treatment of Kidney Stone Disease. Basel, Switzerland: S Karager; 1982

[57] Sass W, Braunlich M, Dreyer H-P, et al. The mechanisms of stone disintegration by shock waves. Ultrasound in Medicine & Biology. 1991;**17**:239-243

[58] Eisenmenger W. The mechanisms of stone fragmentation in ESWL. Ultrasound in Medicine & Biology. 2001;**27**:683-693

[59] Holmer NG, Almquist LO, Hertz TG, et al. On the mechanism of kidney-stone disintegration by acoustic shock-waves. Ultrasound in Medicine & Biology. 1991;**17**:479-489

[60] Sapozhnikov OA, Khokhlova VA, Bailey MR, et al. Effect of overpressure and pulse repetition frequency on cavitation in shock wave lithotripsy. The Journal of the Acoustical Society of America. 2002;**112**(3):1183-1195

[61] Snicorius M, Bakavicius A, Cekauskas A, Miglinas M, et al. Factors

influencing extracorporeal shock wave lithotripsy efficiency for optimal patient selection. Wideochir Inne Tech Maloinwazyjne. 2021;**16**(2):409-416 Available from: Pubmed

[62] Wang LJ, Wong YC, Chuang CK, et al. Predictions of outcomes of renal stones after extracorporeal shock wave lithotripsy from stone characteristics determined by unenhanced helical computed tomography: A multivariate analysis. European Radiology. 2005;**15**:2238-2243

[63] Cho KS, Jung HD, Ham WS, et al. Optimal skin-to-stone distance is a positive predictor for successful outcomes in upper ureter calculi following extracorporeal shock wave lithotripsy: A bayesian model averaging approach. PLoS One. 2015;**10**:e0144912

[64] Delacretaz G, Rink K, Pittomvils G, et al. Importance of the implosion of ESWL-induced cavitation bubbles. Ultrasound in Medicine & Biology. 1995;**21**:97-103

[65] Zhong P, Chuong CJ, Preminger GM. Propagation of shock waves in elastic solids caused by cavitation micro jet impact. II: Application in extracorporeal shock wave lithotripsy. The Journal of the Acoustical Society of America. 1993;**94**:29-36

[66] Sturtevant B. Shock wave physics of lithotriptors. In: Smith AD, editor. Smith's Textbook of Endourology. St. Louis: Quality Medical Publishing, Inc.; 1996. pp. 529-552

[67] Pittomvils G, Vandeursen H, Wevers M, et al. The influence of internal stone structure upon the fracture behaviour of urinary calculi. Ultrasound in Medicine & Biology. 1994;**20**:803-810

[68] Williams JC Jr, Saw KC, Paterson RF, et al. Variability of renal stone fragility in shock wave lithotripsy. Urology. 2003;**61**:1092-1096

[69] Zhu S, Cocks FH, Preminger GM, Zhong P. The role of stress waves and cavitation in stone comminution in shock wave lithotripsy. Ultrasound in Medicine & Biology. 2002;**28**:661-671

[70] Ebrahimi F, Wang F. Fracture behavior of urinary stones under compression. Journal of Biomedical Materials Research. 1989;**23**:507-521

[71] Sokolov DL, Bailey MR, Crum LA. Dual-pulse lithotriptor accelerates stone fragmentation and reduces cell lysis in vitro. Ultrasound in Medicine & Biology. 2003;**29**:1045-1052

[72] Huber P, Debus J, Jöchle K, et al. Control of cavitation activity by different shockwave pulsing regimes. Physics in Medicine and Biology. 1999;**44**:1427-1437

[73] Zhong P, Cocks FH, Cionta I, Preminger GM. Controlled, forced collapse of cavitation bubbles for improved stone fragmentation during shock wave lithotripsy. The Journal of Urology. 1997;**158**:2323-2328

[74] Orkisz M, Farchtchian T, Saighi D, et al. Image based renal stone tracking to improve efficacy in extracorporeal lithotripsy. The Journal of Urology. 1998;**160**:1237-1240

[75] Zhou Y, Cocks FH, Preminger GM, et al. Innovation in shock wave lithotripsy technology: Updates in experimental studies. The Journal of Urology. 2004;**172**:1892-1898

[76] Duryea AP, Hall TL, Maxwell AD, et al. Histotripsy erosion of model urinary calculi. Journal of Endourology. 2011;**25**:341-344

[77] Pishalnikov YA, Sapozhnikov OA, Williams JC Jr, et al. Cavitation bubble

cluster activity in the breakage of kidney stones by lithotripter shock waves. Journal of Endourology. 2003;**17**:435-446

[78] May PC, Bailey MR, Harper JD. Ultrasonic propulsion of kidney stones. Current Opinion in Urology. 2016;**26**(3):264-270

[79] Raskolnikov D, Bailey MR, Harper JD. Recent advances in the science of burst wave lithotripsy and ultrasonic propulsion. BME Frontiers. 2022;**2022**:1-6. DOI: 10.34133/2022/9847952

[80] Zwaschka TA, Ahn JS, Cunitz BW, et al. Combined burst wave lithotripsy and ultrasonic propulsion for improved urinary stone fragmentation. Journal of Endourology. 2018;**32**(4):344-349 Available from: Pubmed

[81] Kim G, Hunter C, Maxwell A, Cunitz BW, et al. Effect of pulse duration and repetition rate on burst wave lithotripsy stone fragmentation in vitro. The Journal of the Acoustical Society of America. 2021;**150**(4):A332 Available from: Pubmed

[82] López-Ramos H, Chavarriaga J, Fakih N. Laser lithotripsy fundamentals: From the physics to optimal fragmentation. International Journal of Innovative Surgery. 2021;**4**(1):1020

[83] Chan KF, Pfefer TJ, Teichman JMH, Welch AJ. A perspective on laser lithotripsy: The fragmentation processes. Journal of Endourology. 2001;**15**:257-273

[84] Peng Q, Juzeniene A, Chen J, Svaasand LO. Lasers in Medicine. Reports on Progress in Physics. 2008;**71**(5):056701

[85] Lee H, Ryan RT, Kim J, Choi B, Arakeri NV, et al. Dependence of calculus retropulsion dynamics on fiber size and radiant exposure during Ho:YAG lithotripsy. Journal of Biomechanical Engineering. 2004;**126**:506-515

[86] Kronenberg P, Traxer O. The laser of the future: Reality and expectations about the new thulium fiber laser- a systematic review. Translational Andrology and Urology. 2019;**8**:S398-S417

[87] Wezel F, Michel MS, Bach T. Effect of pulse energy, Frequency and Length on Holmium: Yttrium-Aluminum-Garnet Laser Fragmentation Efficiency in Non-Floating Artificial Urinary Calculi. Journal of Endourology. 2010;**24**:1135-1140

[88] Patel AP, Knudsen BE. Optimizing use of the holmium: YAG laser for surgical Management of Urinary Lithiasis. Current Urology Reports. 2014;**15**(4):1-7

[89] Fried NM, Irby PB. Advances in laser technology and fibre-optic delivery systems in lithotripsy. Nature Reviews. Urology. 2018;**15**:563-573

[90] Matlaga BR, Chew B, Eisner B, Humphreys M, Knudsen B, Krambeck A, et al. Ureteroscopic laser lithotripsy: A review of dusting vs fragmentation with extraction. Journal of Endourology. 2018;**32**:1-6

[91] Hutchens TC, Blackmon RL, Irby PB, Fried NM. Hollow steel tips for reducing distal fiber burn-back during thulium fiber laser lithotripsy. Journal of Biomedical Optics. 2013;**18**:078001

[92] Blackmon RL, Irby PB, Fried NM. Thulium fiber laser lithotripsy using tapered fibers. Lasers in Surgery and Medicine. 2010;**42**:45-50

[93] Li R, Ruckle D, Keheila M, Maldonado J, Lightfoot M, Alsyouf M, et al. High-frequency dusting versus

conventional holmium laser lithotripsy for intrarenal and ureteral calculi. Journal of Endourology. 2017;**31**:272-277

[94] Elhilali MM, Badaan S, Ibrahim A, Andonian S. Use of the Moses Technology to improve holmium laser lithotripsy outcomes: A preclinical study. Journal of Endourology. 2017;**31**:598-604

[95] Sroka R, Pongratz T, Scheib G, Khoder W, Stief CG, et al. Impact of pulse duration on Ho:YAG laser lithotripsy: Treatment aspects on the single-pulse level. World Journal of Urology. 2015;**33**:479-485

[96] Aldoukhi AH, Roberts WW, Hall TL, Ghani KR. Holmium laser lithotripsy in the new stone age: Dust or bust? Frontiers in Surgery. 2017;**4**:1-6

[97] Aldoukhi AH, Black KM, Ghani KR. Emerging laser techniques for the Management of Stones. The Urologic Clinics of North America. 2019;**46**:193-205

[98] Schatloff O, Lindner U, Ramon J, Winkler HZ. Randomized trial of stone fragment active retrieval versus spontaneous passage during holmium laser lithotripsy for ureteral stones. The Journal of Urology. 2010;**183**:1031-1036

[99] Humphreys MR, Shah OD, Monga M, Chang YH, Krambeck AE, et al. Dusting versus Basketing during Ureteroscopy–which technique is more efficacious?. A prospective multicenter trial from the EDGE research consortium. The Journal of Urology [Internet]. 2018;**199**:1272-1276

[100] Khoder WY, Bader M, Sroka R, Stief C, Waidelich R. Efficacy and safety of Ho:YAG laser lithotripsy for ureteroscopic removal of proximal and distal ureteral calculi. BMC Urology. 2014;**14**:1-7

[101] Noureldin YA, Kallidonis P, Liatsikos EN. Lasers for stone treatment: How safe are they? Current Opinion in Urology. 2020;**30**:130-134

[102] Althunayan AM, Elkoushy MA, Elhilali MM, Andonian S. Adverse events resulting from lasers used in urology. Journal of Endourology. 2014;**28**:256-260

[103] Hardy LA, Kennedy JD, Wilson CR, Irby PB, Fried NM. Cavitation bubble dynamics during thulium fiber laser lithotripsy. Photonic Ther Diagnostics XII. 2016;**9689**:96891B

[104] Patel SR, Nakada SY. The modern history and evolution of percutaneous nephrolithotomy. Journal of Endourology. 2015;**29**(2):153-157

[105] Smith JA, Howards SS, Preminger GM, Dmochowski RR. Hinman's atlas of urologic surgery E-book. Elsevier Health Sciences. 2016

[106] Srisubat A, Potisat S, Lojanapiwat B, Setthawong V, Laopaiboon M. Extracorporeal shock wave lithotripsy (ESWL) versus percutaneous nephrolithotomy (PCNL) or retrograde intrarenal surgery (RIRS) for kidney stones. Cochrane Database of Systematic Reviews. 2014;(11):CD007044

[107] De S, Autorino R, Kim FJ, Zargar H, Laydner H, Balsamo R, et al. Percutaneous nephrolithotomy versus retrograde intrarenal surgery: A systematic review and meta-analysis. European Urology. 2015;**67**(1):125-137

[108] Said SH, Hassan MAAK, Ali RH, Aghaways I, Kakamad FH, Mohammad KQ. Percutaneous nephrolithotomy; alarming variables for postoperative bleeding. Arab Journal of Urology. 2017;**15**(1):24-29

[109] Arora AM, Pawar PW, Tamhankar AS, Sawant AS, Mundhe ST,

Patil SR. Predictors for severe hemorrhage requiring angioembolization post percutaneous nephrolithotomy: A single-center experience over 3 years. Urology Annals. 2019;**11**(2):180

[110] Lee JK, Kim BS, Park YK. Predictive factors for bleeding during percutaneous nephrolithotomy. Korean Journal of Urology. 2013;**54**(7):448-453

[111] Agarwal M, Agrawal MS, Jaiswal A, Kumar D, Yadav H, Lavania P. Safety and efficacy of ultrasonography as an adjunct to fluoroscopy for renal access in percutaneous nephrolithotomy (PCNL). BJU International. 2011;**108**(8):1346-1349

[112] Lahme S, Bichler K-H, Strohmaier WL, Götz T. Minimally invasive PCNL in patients with renal pelvic and calyceal stones. European Urology. 2001;**40**(6):619-624

[113] Xue W, Pacik D, Boellaard W, Breda A, Botoca M, Rassweiler J, et al. Management of single large nonstaghorn renal stones in the CROES PCNL global study. The Journal of Urology. 2012;**187**(4):1293-1297

[114] Rana AM, Bhojwani JP, Junejo NN, Bhagia SD. Tubeless PCNL with patient in supine position: Procedure for all seasons?—With comprehensive technique. Urology. 2008;**71**(4):581-585

[115] Scoffone CM, Cracco CM, Cossu M, Grande S, Poggio M, Scarpa RM. Endoscopic combined intrarenal surgery in Galdakao-modified supine Valdivia position: A new standard for percutaneous nephrolithotomy? European Urology. 2008;**54**(6):1393-1403

[116] Cracco CM, Scoffone CM. Endoscopic combined intrarenal surgery (ECIRS)-tips and tricks to improve outcomes: A systematic review. Turkish Journal of Urology. 2020;**46**(Suppl 1):S46

[117] De La Rosette JJ, Opondo D, Daels FP, Giusti G, Serrano A, Kandasami SV, et al. Categorisation of complications and validation of the Clavien score for percutaneous nephrolithotomy. European Urology. 2012;**62**(2):246-255

[118] Taylor E, Miller J, Chi T, Stoller ML. Complications associated with percutaneous nephrolithotomy. Translational Andrology and Urology. 2012;**1**(4):223

[119] Gok A, Cift A. Predictive factors for bleeding that require a blood transfusion after percutaneous nephrolithotomy. International Journal of Clinical and Experimental Medicine. 2017;**10**(9):13772-13777

[120] Yesil S, Ozturk U, Goktug HNG, Tuygun C, Nalbant I, Imamoglu MA. Previous open renal surgery increased vascular complications in percutaneous nephrolithotomy (PCNL) compared with primary and secondary PCNL and extracorporeal shock wave lithotripsy patients: A retrospective study. Urologia Internationalis. 2013;**91**(3):331-334

[121] Du N, Ma J-Q, Luo J-J, Liu Q-X, Zhang Z-H, Yang M-J, et al. The efficacy and safety of transcatheter arterial embolization to treat renal hemorrhage after percutaneous nephrolithotomy. BioMed Research International. 2019;**2019**:1-10

Chapter 3

Guideline Based Algorithmic Approach for the Management of Renal and Ureteric Calculi

Anshuman Singh, Milap Shah and B.M. Zeeshan Hameed

Abstract

Urolithiasis is a global pathology with increasing prevalence rate. The surgical management of kidney and ureteral stones is based on the stone location, size, the patient's preference and the institutional availability of various modalities. To date, the available modalities in the management of urolithiasis includes external shock wave lithotripsy (ESWL), percutaneous nephrolithotomy (PNL), ureterorenoscopy (URS) including flexible and semirigid ureteroscopy. Tremendous technological advancement in the urological armamentarium has happened since its inception leading to multiple acceptable modalities for the treatment of a particular stone. In accordance with the available recommendations from various institutions and the newer evidence we recommend that the initial choice of modality for the treatment of a renal calculus depends on the stone size and whether the location is lower pole or not. For lower pole stones upto 20 mm PNL and RIRS is efficient irrespective of location while ESWL should only be considered for lower pole stones upto 10 mm. For stones larger than 20 mm mini PNL is effective for stones upto 40 mm while RIRS holds acceptable efficiency for stones not larger than 30 mm. For stones larger than 40 mm standard PNL only should be considered if single stage treatment is attempted.

Keywords: PNL, nephrolithiasis, urolithiasis, SWL, RIRS, URS

1. Introduction

Urolithiasis is a common urinary tract condition with a prevalence of approximately 14% [1]. There are multiple factors which influence an individual's propensity for formation of urinary tract calculi, the most common of which are age, sex, and ethnicity [1, 2]. Anatomically they can have origin in the upper tract or the lower tract of which those originating in the upper tracts are more common while approximately 5% are found within the bladder [3]. They present a significant clinical and economic burden to the healthcare systems [4, 5]. In an attempt to bring uniformity in management worldwide, many institutions have developed extensive guidelines to aid in the evaluation and management of urolithiasis.

Once the diagnosis of urolithiasis is confirmed, the goal of a diagnostic evaluation is to identify, efficiently and economically, the differences present in the patient's metabolic physiology to guide effective preventive strategies for recurrence and

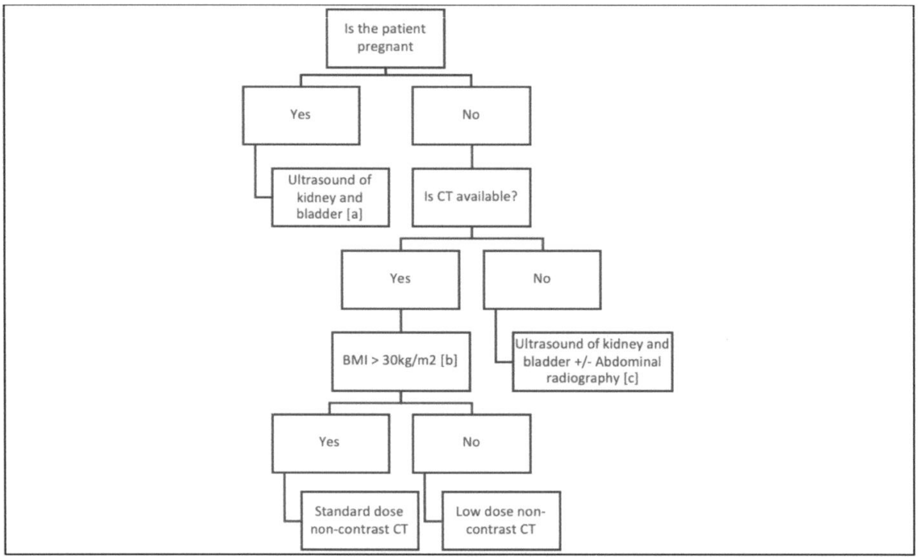

a) For pregnant patients in the third trimester who have intractable pain or fever and in whom the results of an ultrasound of the kidneys and bladder are inadequate, a low-dose, noncontrast CT under guidance of an obstetrician can also be considered to detect suspected nephrolithiasis.
b) In patients with obesity (BMI >30 kg/m^2), standard-dose CT is preferred since low-dose CT may be less reliable for detecting small stones (<2 mm) and ureteral stones.
c) Ultrasound reliably detects hydronephrosis, and radiography can be used to measure stone size and location. However, compared with CT, both ultrasound and radiography are less sensitive for detecting stones.

Figure 1.
A stepwise approach for the diagnostic evaluation of suspected nephrolithiasis.

better assessment of prognosis. The extent of evaluation depends on the factors like: severity and type of stone disease; new stone formation or recurrent stone formation; co-existence of any systemic disease and/or risk factors for recurrent stone formation; family history of nephrolithiasis and last but not the least patient's interest in stone prevention (**Figure 1**).

Technological advancements in the endourological armamentarium have happened at a rapid pace since its inception and is still going on. As a result, the search for the *best* treatment modality for any given stone undergoes a frequent shift from one modality to other in accordance with the newer available evidence. The aim of this chapter is to highlight and summarize in the form of an algorithmic approach the best possible treatment of renal and ureteric calculi in accordance with the recommendations from various urological institutions worldwide along with the newer available evidence.

2. Evaluation of suspected nephrolithiasis

The entire diagnostic workup can be broadly categorized into two categories viz. biochemical and systemic assessment by various laboratory parameters and secondly, imaging specific to nephrolithiasis which will aid in treatment planning [6].

2.1 Biochemical and systemic evaluation

The main aim of biochemical evaluation is identification of any systemic adverse effects secondary to the urinary tract calculi along with a baseline workup of patient as a part of preparation for definitive surgical therapy. This baseline assessment should include evaluation of basic hematological parameters, renal function, urinalysis along with an abbreviated metabolic workup for hypercalcemia, hyperuricemia and hyperphosphatemia. Every attempt should be made to diagnose and treat any urinary tract infection (UTI) prior to definitive surgical therapy to avoid the risk of urosepsis [7].

2.2 Diagnostic imaging

The aim of diagnostic imaging is to confirm the presence of urinary tract calculi and to guide the decision making for the specific modality to be undertaken for treatment. Factors that influence the choice of treatment modality include stone size, location, density and composition, condition of contralateral kidney and presence or absence of complications of stone disease.

2.3 Selection of modality

CT of the abdomen and pelvis without contrast performed using low-radiation-dose protocols is that the gold standard imaging modality for adults with suspected urinary tract calculi, if not contraindicated. In the case of unavailability of CT scan, ultrasonography of the kidneys and bladder in combination with abdominopelvic radiography should be performed [8]. However, in the presence of small radiolucent stones there will be high fraction of stones that will miss the diagnosis. Other imaging modalities like intravenous urography (IVU) and magnetic resonance imaging (MRI) are not preferred as first line investigations and have specific and limited indications.

CT scan also accurately describes stone size and location for treatment planning as it also provides accurate information on the size and number of other stones in the kidneys. If available, there are very few contraindications to perform a low-dose CT [9, 10].

- If the patient is pregnant, an ultrasound is the preferred modality and CT is contraindicated because of risk of teratogenicity to the developing fetus.

- If the patient has a body mass index (BMI) >30 kg/m^2, then a standard-dose CT is preferred because of better exposure.

Computed tomography (CT) of the abdomen and pelvis without contrast reliably detects hydronephrosis and demonstrates the best diagnostic performance for nephrolithiasis. Sensitivity and specificity of CT for detecting ureteral calculi, using conventional radiation doses is, greater than 94% and 97% respectively [11–14]. CT done using low dose protocols is also highly sensitive and specific for detection of >2 mm calculi with a sensitivity and specificity of 97% and 95% respectively [9, 11, 12, 15–17]. Low-dose CT may be less reliable for detecting small stones (<2 mm) and ureteral stones in patients with obesity (BMI >30 mg/k^2). Patients with urolithiasis are at increased risk of recurrent stone formation and also may require repeat imaging sessions. Therefore, low dose CT, if not contraindicated, should be the standard of care to minimize the cumulative radiation exposure to the patients as the sensitivity for detection of stones >3 mm is high and comparable to the standard dose CT in non-obese patients [18, 19]. For the estimation of stone size, low and standard dose CT yield equivalent measurements [20].

3. Surgical treatment of nephrolithiasis

3.1 Goals of surgical therapy

As a part of shared decision making as recommended by American Urology Association, the following factors should be discussed and explained to the patients and the choice of surgical modalities should be made keeping the following factors into consideration along with the patients' preferences.

3.1.1 Stone clearance

Treatment success for ureteral or kidney stone surgery is generally defined in terms of stone clearance rates. Although the definition successful stone clearance is not having unanimous acceptance globally, the absence of residual stones or the presence of residual stone fragments ≤4 mm in size are generally considered a successful outcome. Achieving a stone-free status is important, since small residual stone fragments, particularly those >4 mm, may act as a nidus leading to aggregation and recurrent stone formation. Many centres also evaluate the need for re-treatment or additional procedures for complete stone clearance and consider it as another important measure of efficacy of any modality of treatment.

3.1.2 Risk of adverse events

The benefits of surgical stone removal must be balanced against the risk for adverse events and complications. Procedures that offer the highest stone clearance rates (such as ureteroscopy [URS] and percutaneous nephrolithotomy [PNL]) are also believed to have higher complication rates. The decision making should incorporate a detailed discussion with the patient regarding the possible adverse events and the subsequent need for ancillary treatments.

3.1.3 Effect on quality of life (QoL)

The treatment planning should also take into account the patients' perspective regarding the treatment and the subsequent overall impact on patient's quality of life depending upon factors like patient's perception of pain and other discomforting symptoms, the total number of hospital visits and admissions and the overall healthcare related economic impact on the patient.

4. Choice of surgical approach

The factors that play a role in the selection of a modality for surgical treatment of nephrolithiasis can be divided into patient factors (comorbidities, body habitus, pregnancy, infection, bleeding diathesis and patient preference) and factors related to the stone like size, location and composition of stone. Choice of the treatment modality should be a part of shared decision making between the patient and the healthcare provider. However, it can broadly be classified into two categories depending on whether the indication of procedure is emergency or a planned intervention.

4.1 Emergency surgery

Urgent decompression of the collecting system with either PNL or ureteroscopy (URS) with urinary diversion should be done if UTI is ruled out and emergency intervention is indicated [21]. On the other hand, in the presence of suspected or confirmed UTI urgent drainage of the collecting system by a ureteral stent or percutaneous nephrostomy tube should be instituted along with empirical antimicrobial therapy till urinary culture specific antibiotics can be instituted. Definitive stone management should be done once the infection is treated because stone manipulation in the presence of active UTI may lead to life-threatening urosepsis and should therefore be avoided [22]. Mortality has been found to be lower in patients who are treated with urgent surgical decompression followed by delayed definitive management compared with those who are taken up for upfront definitive treatment and lack of surgical decompression [22]. There is no specific recommendation regarding the choice of modality for urinary diversion as both the modalities, i.e. indwelling double J stents and percutaneous nephrostomy tubes, have been shown to be equally effective at drainage in one randomized trial [21].

4.2 Elective surgery

Ureteral stones — If emergency management of ureteric stones is not required, the choice of treatment modality for planned removal of stone depends upon stone factors, anatomical factors and patient factors [7]. Stone factors include the total stone size and total stone burden, location of stones and the density of stones (assessed by the Hounsfield units of the stone). Anatomical factors include the urinary tract anatomy, presence of any distal obstruction or any congenital anatomical anomaly. Patient factors include the factors like pregnancy, bleeding diathesis and obesity.

For proximal and mid-ureteric stones ≤10 mm, SWL or URS is the most commonly performed procedure. For >10 mm stones in the same location, SWL is not recommended and URS is considered the first-line therapy. For **distal ureteric** stones, irrespective of the size, URS is considered the first-line treatment option. SWL is not suitable in patients with obesity, pregnancy, uncontrolled bleeding diathesis, abnormal urinary tract anatomy, and in stones with high attenuation (i.e., >900 Hounsfield units on preoperative CT scan). PNL, laparoscopic, robot-assisted, and open surgery are generally reserved for patients in whom SWL and/or URS are unsuccessful, or in patients with a complex kidney or ureteral anatomy. However, in patients who are planned to undergo concomitant open or reconstructive surgery for coexisting anatomical anomalies (e.g., ureteropelvic junction [UPJ] obstruction or ureteral stricture), the procedure can be combined with stone retrieval prior to reconstruction.

The rationale for this above mentioned approach is based on the results of multiple meta-analyses of randomized trials that have shown that URS offers higher stone-free rates (SFRs) and requires fewer retreatments and secondary procedures as compared to SWL, but with a higher rate of complications [23–27]. A 2016 systematic review that evaluated the efficacy of URS and SWL for the treatment of ureteral stones reported that the overall SFR with URS is significantly greater than that with SWL [23]. This difference in SFR with URS was also noted for subgroup of patients with stones ≤10 mm at all locations in the ureter and also for stones >10 mm in mid and distal ureter. For stones >10 mm in the proximal ureter, SFR was comparable between URS and SWL [23]. Complication rates for all the complications were comparable between both the groups except for ureteric perforation which was higher in the URS group [23]. However, another meta-analysis by Aboumarzouk et al. has reported higher procedure related complication rate with URS as compared to SWL [24]. The number of retreatments required with URS is lower than that required with SWL [28].

Kidney stones — SWL, URS, and PNL are the most commonly used surgical modalities for patients with kidney stones. In patients where emergency management of renal calculi is not indicated, modality for elective management is selected based on multiple stone factors, anatomical factors and patient factors as is the case with ureteric stones. Stone factors include the total stone size and total stone burden, location of stones and the density of stones (assessed by the Hounsfield units of the stone). Anatomical factors include the urinary tract anatomy, presence of any distal obstruction or any congenital anatomical anomaly. Patient factors include the factors like pregnancy, bleeding diathesis and obesity.

Traditionally, PNL has been associated with maximum stone clearance with the disadvantage mainly associated to the invasive nature of procedure with risk of hemorrhage. Advancements in technology has focused on minimizing the morbidity associated with PNL by reducing the diameter of sheath size and nephroscopes resulting in lesser invasion of renal parenchyma. This miniaturization has evolved from the first description of minimally invasive techniques by Lahme et al., which used an access sheath with outer diameter of 18F (inner diameter of 15F) and a 12F nephroscope, to the micro-PNL described by Bader et al. which uses a 4.85F "all seeing needle" only along with laser fragmentation and dusting of the stone. Other modifications include ultra-mini PNL first described by Desai et al. using a 11F amplatz and 6F nephroscope and super-mini PNL described by Zeng et al. which uses an active irrigation and suction mechanism attached to a miniaturized PNL system where the fragment evacuation is done by the so called "vacuum cleaner effect" [29].

The current prevalent approach to the choice of surgical modality, largely in accordance with the 2016 American Urological Association/Endourological Society and 2018 European Association of Urology guidelines [23, 30], is as follows:

For ≤20 mm superior calyceal, middle calyceal or pelvic calculi, SWL or URS is the preferred modality while for inferior calyceal stones, URS or PNL is preferred. SWL is not preferred for inferior calyceal stones keeping in mind the poor stone clearance rates of SWL for lower pole stones. For stones that are >20 mm, PNL is considered the first-line option irrespective of the stone location. If PNL is not available or contraindicated, staged URS (i.e., performed in separate planned sessions) can be a viable alternative. The evidence guiding the rationale for this approach is based upon several randomized trials and meta-analyses [23, 31–42]. Collectively, these studies have shown that SFR for both SWL and URS gradually decreases with the increasing stone size, whereas efficacy of PNL in terms of stone clearance is minimally affected with the stone burden [31]. For stones <20 mm located in upper pole, middle calyx, or pelvis of the kidney, SWL and URS offer SFRs of roughly 50 to 80 percent [31, 43]. In a meta-analysis comparing SWL to URS for renal calculi of size 10 to 20 mm, URS provided improved SFR and lower retreatment rate without an increase in complication rates [32]. For lower pole renal calculi URS and PNL offer significantly improved stone clearance rates compared to SWL, with a moderate increase in the rate of complications. These findings are corroborated by the results of a systematic review, for lower pole renal calculi of size 10 to 20 mm, which showed highest SFR for PNL followed by URS and SWL [23]. For stones >20 mm, SFR for SWL was as low as 10 percent [23]. The reason for this reduction in SFR of SWL with increasing stone burden in the lower pole is mainly because of poor clearance of stone fragments post disintegration rand not due to poor efficiency of disintegration which is not much affected by the stone location within the kidney.

5. Evidence based recommendations and comparison of various guidelines regarding choice of surgical procedure: a summary of available guidelines

Recommendations from the American Urological Association guidelines when analyzed in comparison to the guidelines from Canadian Urological Association, European Association of Urology, National Institute for Health and Care Excellence guidelines and Urological Association of Asia revealed a high level of consensus surrounding the medical management of urinary tract calculi [44]. For surgical management, there was noted to be a high level of consensus regarding certain aspects of treatment of ureteral stones, including not pre stenting for uncomplicated ureteroscopy and employment of either ureteroscopy or shockwave lithotripsy as first line treatment. Jiang et al. [44] performed a qualitative review of the available major guidelines on the management of nephrolithiasis and noted a consensus on most of the factors but a discordance was also noted in certain stone categories. Also only UAA guidelines distinguish between the indications for traditional PCNL vs. mini-PCNL, micro-PCNL or ultramini-PCNL. The risk of complications, especially postoperative hemorrhage, after PCNL had traditionally limited its use as a first line surgical option only for bigger calculi (>20 mm) or lower pole calculi >10 mm. However, with the continued technological advancements in endourology and development of miniaturized techniques of PCNL have led to lesser renal parenchymal loss and lesser hemorrhage. The increasing use of these miniaturized PCNL techniques has led to availability of better quality of evidence regarding their safety and efficacy when compared to the other available options like SWL and RIRS. As can be seen in the below mentioned algorithm comparing the recommendations of various guidelines for the choice of modality of surgical treatment of renal calculi, the miniaturized PCNL techniques which are gradually replacing standard PCNL are not taken into consideration (**Figure 2**).

The greatest discordance among various guidelines for the choice of surgical treatment modality can be seen in the upper pole and interpolar calculi of size <10 mm and 10 - 20 mm where the first line options as proposed by various guidelines differ. For upper pole calculi of size upto 10 mm SWL is the recommended modality by NICE guidelines while AUA and EAU guidelines recommend for URS or SWL for stones upto 20 mm. UAA guidelines, on the other hand, take into account the newer miniaturized options of ultra-mini or micro PCNL and recommend it to be the modality of choice for stones upto 20 mm. For stones larger than 20 mm all guidelines unanimously recommend for PCNL irrespective of stone location. Discordance in recommendations is also seen for lower pole stones of size 10-20 mm and in this regard, the AUA appears to favor the use of PCNL but does not necessarily mandate its use over RIRS [23]. Instead, they insist that patients should be informed about the improved SFR of PCNL with increased risk of adverse events. On the other hand, the EAU guidelines very clearly recommend the use of PNL for lower pole calculi >20 mm and suggest that it should be *highly considered* for stones in the 10 - 20 mm range as well (**Table 1**) [45]. These recommendations have not specifically mentioned about the use of mini, ultra-mini or super mini PCNL (**Figure 2**).

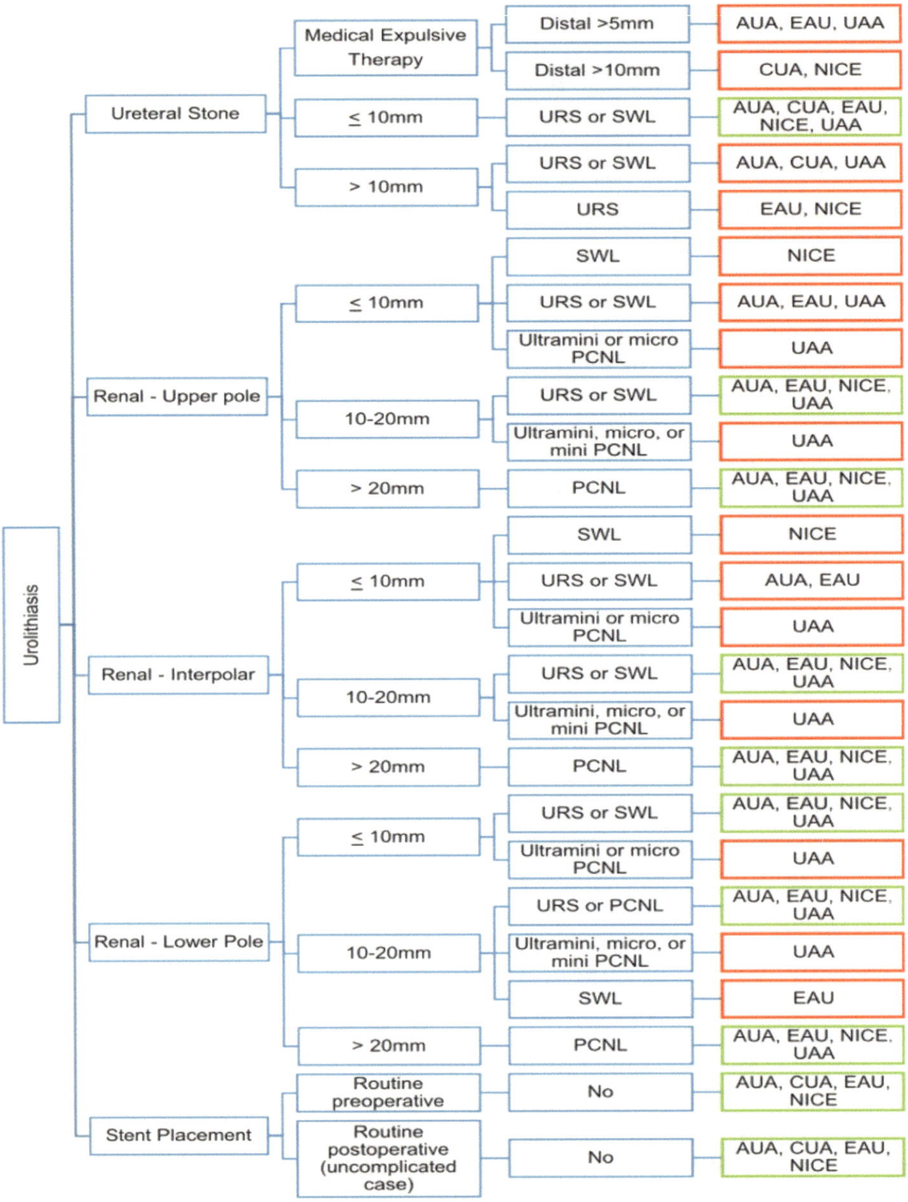

Abbreviations used in Figure 2	
AUA [American Urological Association]	NICE [National Institute for Health and Care Excellence]
CT [Computerized Tomography]	PCNL [Percutaneous Nephrolithotomy]
CUA [Canadian Urological Association]	SWL [Shockwave Lithotripsy]
EAU [European Association of Urology]	UAA [Urological Association of Asia]

Figure 2.
Comparative description of recommendations of various guidelines for selection of modality for surgical management of nephrolithiasis [44].

Guideline	Stone size	SWL	RIRS	PNL
AUA	10 mm	Preferred	Preferred	Discouraged
	10-20 mm	Discouraged	Allowed	Preferred
	>20 mm	Discouraged	Allowed	Preferred
EAU	10 mm	Preferred	Preferred	Discouraged
	10-20 mm	Allowed	Allowed	Allowed
	>20 mm	Discouraged	Discouraged	Preferred

Table 1.
Recommendations for the surgical management of lower pole stones based on current AUA and EAU guidelines.

A meta-analysis of randomized controlled trials by Feng et al. [46] concluded that mPCNL had a higher SFR than standard PCNL and there was no significant difference between the two groups regarding ≥2 cm renal calculi. Besides, mPCNL has been noted to be associated with significantly less bleeding and a lower transfusion rate. Further, a multi-institutional comparative study by Liu et al. [47] showed SMP to be safe and highly effective for renal calculi upto 4 cm with lesser postoperative complications as compared to standard PCNL. However, for stones larger than 4 cm the stone clearance by SMP was lower than standard PCNL. The better efficacy of mini PNL in terms of stone free rates and improved stone clearance has been corroborated by a recent network meta-analysis of randomized trials by Tsai et al. [48] Another network meta-analysis by Chungh et al. [49] comparing PCNL, RIRS and SWL showed PCNL to have the maximum stone free rates followed by RIRS. SWL was shown to have the least stone free rates. Subgroup analysis for lower pole stones showed similar results. Complications (in SWL, PCNL, and RIRS were 12.5%, 20.2%, and 15.0%, respectively) were greater in the patients undergoing PCNL but the major complications (15.4% in SWL, 13.8% in PCNL, and 18.3% in RIRS) were comparable between the three groups.

6. PCNL as a day-care procedure?

PNL is traditionally conducted as a procedure that necessitates hospitalization rather than outpatient care. However, there is significant pressure to use health care resources as effectively as possible in order to continuously improve medical quality and patient satisfaction with as little medical expenditure as possible. This attempt for optimal utilization of hospital resources, particularly in the publicly funded health care system, is one of the primary indications to attempt to cut down the costs associated with the hospitalization required for PCNL. Complications after PCNL and the length of hospital stay have already been steadily declining mainly attributable to the less invasive approaches and advancements in postoperative pain management [50]. Discharging the day of procedure or no later than 24 hours following surgery is referred to as day-care PCNL [51–53] and is regarded as a potential viable option for some patients, supported by emerging evidence [51–55]. Grade I and II complications following PCNL are the most common and may usually be managed conservatively or in a brief course [56]. The early studies were conducted on tiny cohorts, and in 2005,

Singh et al. published their initial findings on a small series of the day-care PCNL that included 10 patients. The reported readmission rates for day-care PCNL have ranged from 0 to 10% [51]. Jones et al. conducted a systematic review on the safety and efficacy of day-care PNL and concluded that it is a safe procedure when preoperative preparation and patient selection are done judiciously [51]. However, there still is a lot of concern about patient safety, which keeps this approach from being incorporated into routine practice. Furthermore, there aren't many research that compare day-care and inpatient results and formal cost-effectiveness assessments. There is still lack of good quality evidence which comprehensively evaluates the safety and efficacy of day-care PCNL along with the advantage of cost effectiveness and this gap needs to be bridged before formal incorporation of day-care PCNL for management of renal calculi can be done for global acceptance.

7. Conclusion

We therefore, based on the newer evidences on the miniaturized modifications of PCNL and their comparative analysis with RIRS and SWL, recommend the following approach for the appropriate selection of surgical modality for renal and ureteral calculi.

For renal calculi upto 20 mm, the choice of surgical modality should be based on the stone location. For lower pole stones of size upto 10 mm, super mini or ultra-mini modifications of PCNL can be considered the first line modality because of proven safety and improved efficacy in terms of stone clearance. However, RIRS and SWL can also be considered in case of unavailability of SMP or UMP. For lower pole stones of size 10-20 mm, SMP or UMP should be preferred if available due to the already mentioned factors. SWL for stones 10–20 mm in lower pole should be avoided given the increased propensity of requirement of repeat procedure due to poor stone clearance in one session.

For renal calculi of size greater than 20 mm, decision should be made depending on further stratifying the stone size of less than 4 cm or more than 4 cm. Stones up to 4 cm can be efficiently cleared by miniaturized PCNL and therefore it should be the

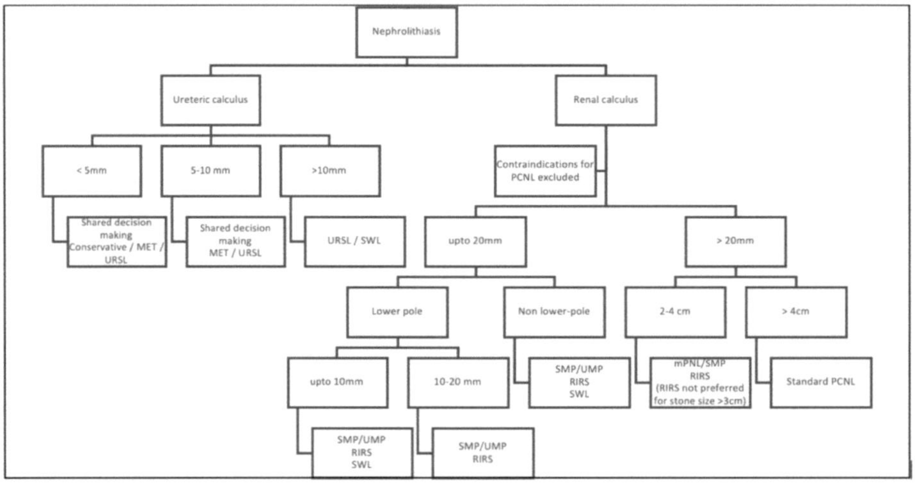

Figure 3.
Approach for surgical management of nephrolithiasis.

preferred modality due to improved safety profile as compared to standard PCNL. However for stones larger than 4 cm, the clearance has been sub-optimal using miniaturized techniques and standard PCNL should be the preferred approach (**Figure 3**).

As is easily understood by the discussion, the technical advancements and miniaturization of PCNL is leading to its increased use and applicability to the various domains which were previously being primarily managed by other less invasive modalities like RIRS and SWL. Given its increasing safety profile and comparable efficacy to standard PCNL, it can now be used for almost all stone categories except for very large stones without the risk of significant complications and therefore is becoming a promising modality to replace the standard PCNL as the gold standard modality for treatment of nephrolithiasis.

Conflict of interest

None.

Notes/thanks/other declarations

None.

Acronyms and abbreviations

CT	Computerized Tomography
IVP	Intravenous Pyelography
MRI	Magnetic Resonance Imaging
BMI	Body Mass Index
CI	Confidence Interval
SFR	Stone Free Rate
PNL	Percutaneous Nephrolithotomy
URS	Ureterorenoscopy
UTI	Urinary Tract Infection
SWL	Shockwave Lithotripsy
UPJ	Ureteropelvic Junction
AUA	American Urological Association
CUA	Canadian Urological Association
EAU	European Association of Urology
NICE	National Institute for Health and Care Excellence

Author details

Anshuman Singh[1], Milap Shah[2] and B.M. Zeeshan Hameed[3]*

1 Department of Urology, Manipal Academy of Higher Education, Manipal, India

2 Department of Urology, Max Hospitals, Saket, New Delhi, India

3 Department of Urology, Father Mueller Medical College, Mangalore, India

*Address all correspondence to: zeeshanhameedbm@gmail.com

References

[1] Curhan GC. Epidemiology of stone disease. The Urologic Clinics of North America. 2007;**34**:287-293

[2] Rukin NJ, Siddiqui ZA, Chedgy ECP, Somani BK. Trends in up- per tract stone disease in England: Evidence from the hospital epi- sodes statistics database. Urologia Internationalis. 2017;**98**:391-396

[3] Schwartz BF, Stoller ML. The vesical calculus. The Urologic Clinics of North America. 2000;**27**:333-346

[4] Geraghty RM, Jones P, Hermann TRW, Aboumarkzouk O, Somani BK. Ureteroscopy is more cost effective than shock wave litho- tripsy for stone treatment: Systematic review and meta-analysis. World Journal of Urology. 2018;**36**:1783-1793

[5] Geraghty RM, Cook P, Walker V, Somani BK. Evaluation of the economic burden of kidney stone disease in the UK: A retrospec- tive cohort study with a mean follow-up of 19 years. BJU International. 2020;**125**:586-594

[6] Pak CY, Britton F, Peterson R, et al. Ambulatory evaluation of nephrolithiasis. Classification, clinical presentation and diagnostic criteria. The American Journal of Medicine. 1980;**69**(1):19-30

[7] Wang CJ, Hsu CS, Chen HW, Chang CH, Tsai PC. Percutaneous nephrostomy versus ureteroscopic management of sepsis associated with ureteral stone impaction: A randomized controlled trial. Urolithiasis. Oct 2016;**44**(5):415-419. DOI: 10.1007/s00240-015-0852-7. Epub 2015 Dec 11. PMID: 26662171

[8] Ulusan S, Koc Z, Tokmak N. Accuracy of sonography for detecting renal stone: Comparison with CT. Journal of Clinical Ultrasound. 2007;**35**:256

[9] Niemann T, Kollmann T, Bongartz G. Diagnostic performance of low-dose CT for the detection of urolithiasis: A meta-analysis. AJR. American Journal of Roentgenology. 2008;**191**:396

[10] Jung SI, Kim YJ, Park HS, et al. Sensitivity of digital abdominal radiography for the detection of ureter stones by stone size and location. Journal of Computer Assisted Tomography. 2010;**34**:879

[11] Fulgham PF, Assimos DG, Pearle MS, Preminger GM. Clinical effectiveness protocols for imaging in the management of ureteral calculous disease: AUA technology assessment. The Journal of Urology. 2013;**189**:1203

[12] Pfister SA, Deckart A, Laschke S, et al. Unenhanced helical computed tomography vs intravenous urography in patients with acute flank pain: Accuracy and economic impact in a randomized prospective trial. European Radiology. 2003;**13**:2513

[13] Smith RC, Verga M, McCarthy S, Rosenfield AT. Diagnosis of acute flank pain: Value of unenhanced helical CT. AJR. American Journal of Roentgenology. 1996;**166**:97

[14] Ulahannan D, Blakeley CJ, Jeyadevan N, Hashemi K. Benefits of CT urography in patients presenting to the emergency department with suspected ureteric colic. Emergency Medicine Journal. 2008;**25**:569

[15] Kim BS, Hwang IK, Choi YW, et al. Low-dose and standard-dose unenhanced helical computed

tomography for the assessment of acute renal colic: Prospective comparative study. Acta Radiologica. 2005;**46**:756

[16] Liu W, Esler SJ, Kenny BJ, et al. Low-dose nonenhanced helical CT of renal colic: Assessment of ureteric stone detection and measurement of effective dose equivalent. Radiology. 2000;**215**:51

[17] Tack D, Sourtzis S, Delpierre I, et al. Low-dose unenhanced multidetector CT of patients with suspected renal colic. AJR. American Journal of Roentgenology. 2003;**180**:305

[18] Ciaschini MW, Remer EM, Baker ME, et al. Urinary calculi: Radiation dose reduction of 50% and 75% at CT--effect on sensitivity. Radiology. 2009;**251**:105

[19] Poletti PA, Platon A, Rutschmann OT, et al. Low-dose versus standard-dose CT protocol in patients with clinically suspected renal colic. AJR. American Journal of Roentgenology. 2007;**188**:927

[20] Sohn W, Clayman RV, Lee JY, et al. Low-dose and standard computed tomography scans yield equivalent stone measurements. Urology. 2013;**81**:231

[21] Pearle MS, Pierce HL, Miller GL, et al. Optimal method of urgent decompression of the collecting system for obstruction and infection due to ureteral calculi. The Journal of Urology. 1998;**160**:1260

[22] Borofsky MS, Walter D, Shah O, et al. Surgical decompression is associated with decreased mortality in patients with sepsis and ureteral calculi. The Journal of Urology. 2013;**189**:946

[23] Assimos D, Krambeck A, Miller NL, et al. Surgical Management of Stones: American urological association/ Endourological society guideline, PART II. The Journal of Urology. 2016;**196**:1161

[24] Aboumarzouk OM, Kata SG, Keeley FX, McClinton S, Nabi G. Extracorporeal shock wave lithotripsy (ESWL) versus ureteroscopic management for ureteric calculi. Cochrane Database of Systematic Reviews. May 2012;**16**(5):CD006029. DOI: 10.1002/14651858.CD006029.pub4. PMID: 22592707

[25] Matlaga BR, Jansen JP, Meckley LM, et al. Treatment of ureteral and renal stones: A systematic review and meta-analysis of randomized, controlled trials. The Journal of Urology. 2012;**188**:130

[26] Cui X, Ji F, Yan H, et al. Comparison between extracorporeal shock wave lithotripsy and ureteroscopic lithotripsy for treating large proximal ureteral stones: A meta-analysis. Urology. 2015;**85**:748

[27] Drake T, Grivas N, Dabestani S, et al. What are the benefits and harms of Ureteroscopy compared with shock-wave lithotripsy in the treatment of upper ureteral stones? A systematic review. European Urology. 2017;**72**:772

[28] Preminger GM, Tiselius HG, Assimos DG, et al. 2007 guideline for the management of ureteral calculi. The Journal of Urology. 2007;**178**:2418

[29] Lahme S. Miniaturisation of PCNL. Urolithiasis. 2018;**46**(1):99-106. DOI: 10.1007/s00240-017-1029-3

[30] http://uroweb.org/guideline/urolithiasis/

[31] Srisubat A, Potisat S, Lojanapiwat B, Setthawong V, Laopaiboon M. Extracorporeal shock wave lithotripsy (ESWL) versus percutaneous nephrolithotomy (PCNL) or retrograde

intrarenal surgery (RIRS) for kidney stones. Cochrane Database of Systematic Reviews. Nov 2014;**24**(11):CD007044. DOI: 10.1002/14651858.CD007044.pub3. PMID: 25418417

[32] Pearle MS, Lingeman JE, Leveillee R, et al. Prospective, randomized trial comparing shock wave lithotripsy and ureteroscopy for lower pole caliceal calculi 1 cm or less. The Journal of Urology. 2005;**173**:2005

[33] Preminger GM. Management of lower pole renal calculi: Shock wave lithotripsy versus percutaneous nephrolithotomy versus flexible ureteroscopy. Urological Research. 2006;**34**:108

[34] Zheng C, Yang H, Luo J, et al. Extracorporeal shock wave lithotripsy versus retrograde intrarenal surgery for treatment for renal stones 1-2 cm: A meta-analysis. Urolithiasis. 2015;**43**:549

[35] Karakoyunlu N, Goktug G, Şener NC, et al. A comparison of standard PNL and staged retrograde FURS in pelvis stones over 2 cm in diameter: A prospective randomized study. Urolithiasis. 2015;**43**:283

[36] Zheng C, Xiong B, Wang H, et al. Retrograde intrarenal surgery versus percutaneous nephrolithotomy for treatment of renal stones >2 cm: A meta-analysis. Urologia Internationalis. 2014;**93**:417

[37] Donaldson JF, Lardas M, Scrimgeour D, et al. Systematic review and meta-analysis of the clinical effectiveness of shock wave lithotripsy, retrograde intrarenal surgery, and percutaneous nephrolithotomy for lower-pole renal stones. European Urology. 2015;**67**:612

[38] Kumar A, Kumar N, Vasudeva P, et al. A prospective, randomized comparison of shock wave lithotripsy, retrograde intrarenal surgery and miniperc for treatment of 1 to 2 cm radiolucent lower calyceal renal calculi: A single center experience. The Journal of Urology. 2015;**193**:160

[39] Sener NC, Imamoglu MA, Bas O, et al. Prospective randomized trial comparing shock wave lithotripsy and flexible ureterorenoscopy for lower pole stones smaller than 1 cm. Urolithiasis. 2014;**42**:127

[40] Kumar A, Vasudeva P, Nanda B, et al. A prospective randomized comparison between shock wave lithotripsy and flexible Ureterorenoscopy for lower Caliceal stones ≤2 cm: A single-Center experience. Journal of Endourology. 2015;**29**:575

[41] Mi Y, Ren K, Pan H, et al. Flexible ureterorenoscopy (F-URS) with holmium laser versus extracorporeal shock wave lithotripsy (ESWL) for treatment of renal stone <2 cm: A meta-analysis. Urolithiasis. 2016;**44**:353

[42] Zhang W, Zhou T, Wu T, et al. Retrograde intrarenal surgery versus percutaneous Nephrolithotomy versus extracorporeal shockwave lithotripsy for treatment of lower pole renal stones: A Meta-analysis and systematic review. Journal of Endourology. 2015;**29**:745

[43] Khan SR, Pearle MS, Robertson WG, et al. Kidney stones. Nature Reviews. Disease Primers. 2016;**2**:16008

[44] Jiang P, Xie L, Arada R, Patel RM, Landman J, Clayman RV. Qualitative review of clinical guidelines for medical and surgical Management of Urolithiasis: Consensus and controversy 2020. The Journal of Urology. 2021;**205**(4):999-1008. DOI: 10.1097/JU.0000000000001478

[45] Türk C, Petřík A, Sarica K, Seitz C, Skolarikos A, Straub M, et al. EAU

guidelines on interventional treatment for urolithiasis. European Urology. 2016;**69**:475-482

[46] Feng D, Hu X, Tang Y, Han P, Wei X. The efficacy and safety of miniaturized percutaneous nephrolithotomy versus standard percutaneous nephrolithotomy: A systematic review and meta-analysis of randomized controlled trials. Investigative and Clinical Urology. 2020;**61**(2):115-126. DOI: 10.4111/icu.2020.61.2.115

[47] Liu Y, Cai C, Aquino A, Al-Mousawi S, Zhang X, Choong SKS, et al. Management of large renal stones with super-mini percutaneous nephrolithotomy: An international multicentre comparative study. BJU International. 2020;**126**(1):168-176. DOI: 10.1111/bju.15066

[48] Tsai SH, Chung HJ, Tseng PT, Wu YC, Tu YK, Hsu CW, et al. Comparison of the efficacy and safety of shockwave lithotripsy, retrograde intrarenal surgery, percutaneous nephrolithotomy and minimally invasive percutaneous nephrolithotomy for lower-pole renal stones: A systematic review and network meta-analysis. Medicine. 2020;**99**(10):e19403

[49] Chung DY, Kang DH, Cho KS, Jeong WS, Jung HD, Kwon JK, et al. Comparison of stone-free rates following shock wave lithotripsy, percutaneous nephrolithotomy, and retrograde intrarenal surgery for treatment of renal stones: A systematic review and network meta-analysis. PLoS One. 2019;**14**(2):e0211316. DOI: 10.1371/journal.pone.0211316

[50] Güler A, Erbin A, Ucpinar B, et al. Comparison of minia- turized percutaneous nephrolithotomy and standard percutaneous nephrolithotomy for the treatment of large kidney stones: A ran- domized prospective study. Urolithiasis. 2019;**47**:289-295. DOI: 10.1007/s00240-018-1061-y

[51] Jones P, Bennett G, Dosis A, Pietropaolo A, Geraghty R, Aboumarzouk O, et al. Safety and efficacy of day-case percutaneous nephrolithotomy: a systematic review from european society of uro-technology. European Urology Focus. Nov 2019;**5**(6):1127-1134. DOI: 10.1016/j.euf.2018.04.002. Epub 2018 Apr 12. PMID: 29657068

[52] Schoenfeld D, Zhou T, Stern JM. Outcomes for patients undergoing ambulatory percutaneous nephrolithotomy. Journal of Endourology. 2019;**33**:189-193. DOI: 10.1089/end.2018.0579

[53] Bechis SK, Han DS, Abbott JE, et al. Outpatient percuta- neous nephrolithotomy: The UC san diego health experience. Journal of Endourology. 2018;**32**:394-401. DOI: 10.1089/end.2018.0056

[54] Beiko D, Lee L. Outpatient tubeless percutaneous nephro- lithotomy: The initial case series. Canadian Urological Association Journal. 2010;**4**:E86-E90

[55] Singh I, Kumar A, Kumar P. "Ambulatory PCNL" (tube- less PCNL under regional anesthesia)—A preliminary report of 10 cases. International Urology and Nephrology. 2005;**37**:35-37. DOI: 10.1007/s1125 5-004-6706-9

[56] de la Rosette JJMCH, Opondo D, Daels FPJ, et al. Categorisation of complications and validation of the Clavien score for percutaneous nephrolithotomy. European Urology. 2012;**62**:246-255. DOI: 10.1016/j.eururo.2012.03.055

Chapter 4

Perspective Chapter: Medicinal Plants for the Treatment of Nephrolithiasis

Farah Al-Mamoori and Talal Aburjai

Abstract

Nephrolithiasis (kidney stones) impacts a significant group of individuals today as a result of changing lifestyles. Over the past decade, there has been a revival of interest in the study of medicinal plants as a source of potential herbal medicine. Herbal medicine could become a new phase in the medical system for human disease management within the next few decades. In fact, a number of studies strongly suggest using medicinal herbs as one of the anti-nephrolithiatic treatments. Different bioactive substances found in plants, such as polyphenols, flavonoids, saponins, furanochromones, alkaloids, and terpenoids, may be useful in halting the development of stones. These natural resources do in fact contain bioactive compounds of many types, including phenolic acids, flavonoids, and terpenoids, which have recently been shown to have potent anti-nephrolithiatic properties. However, the outcomes of the experiments that have been conducted with these natural substances are still in the preclinical stages. Future research on clinical applications may therefore be a fruitful way to confirm the clinical utility of these medications.

Keywords: medicinal plants, herbs, kidney stones, nephrolithiasis, flavonoids, phenolic acids

1. Introduction

Nephrolithiasis(kidney stone) is an illness that affects individuals of all sexes, races, and ages and is believed to be on the rise in many countries around the world. Along with the consequences of global warming, eating patterns may be a major factor influencing these trends [1]. Around 12% of people worldwide will get kidney stones at certain time in their lives. Kidney stones raise the risk of developing chronic kidney disease by 60% and end-stage renal disease by 40%, and papillary renal cell carcinoma has also been linked to kidney stones [2].

The utilization of herbal products has recently gained more attention due to the high cost and negative side effects of instrument implantation and urinary tract surgery. Humans and even animals have long relied on medicinal plants as a significant source of food and medicine. Nowadays, a number of researchers base their studies on natural resources such as medicinal herbs and a range of antiquated techniques such as those used by Ibn Sina [3]. Medical plants alleviate kidney stone pain and inhibit lithogenesis. From the kidney, medicinal plants eliminate kidney stones. Kidney stones are frequently treated with medicinal plants (calcium oxalate, uric acid, struvite, and cysteine). The evolution of modern civilization includes the use of herbal medicine [4].

The formation of stones may be avoided by the existence of many bioactive components found in such as polyphenols, flavonoids, phytosterols, saponins, furanochromones, alkaloids, and terpenoids. Evidence points to their potential litholytic, antispasmodic, and diuretic properties as well as an inhibitory influence on crystallization, nucleation, and aggregation of crystals as the possible causes of their therapeutic effects. These benefits may be caused by antioxidant, anti-inflammatory, or antibacterial characteristics, according to the molecular pathways involved [5]. This chapter summarizes the role bioactive compounds and mechanisms of medicinal plants in the treatment of nephrolithiasis.

2. Anti-urolithiatic plants

The various traditionally based groups of medicinal plants have been used as anti-urolithiatic drugs belonging to the families including: Amaranthaceae, Malvaceae, Meliaceae, Satavari, Oxalidaceae, Crassulaceae, Saxifragaceae, etc. Considering the presence of therapeutic activities such as anti-inflammatory, antioxidant, analgesic, diuretic, or lithotriptic activities, these plants have been used as mono or polyherbs in anti-nephrolithiatic formulations [6].

The fruits of the *Rubus idaeus* L. plant, also known as raspberries, are an abundant supply of glycosaminoglycans, citrate, and magnesium that can help prevent kidney stones. Epigallocatechin, a polyphenolic component that is widely distributed in *Camellia sinensis* L. (green tea), has been shown to be effective in treating kidney stones. It works as a potent antioxidant to reduce oxidative stress and the risk of stone development. *Petroselinum crispum* Mill. (parsley) contains large amounts of apiol and myristicin, two compounds with biological properties that are antioxidants and diuretics and are thought to be beneficial in the treatment of urolithiasis. The tree pomegranate, or *Punica granatum* L., is a common name for a fruit that contains active ingredients such as flavonoids, alkaloids, glycosides, and steroids with antioxidant and anti-inflammatory properties [7].

Clinical investigations have mostly focused on finding out if the stone incidence, or the frequency and size of kidney stones, has changed. Large stones shrank while little stones were destroyed. The majority of research found that herbs had diuretic properties. Typically, kidney stones are found in the ureters and renal pelvis. The most likely cause of stone passage and elimination is increased urine volume. It's unknown what led to the size reduction. As a result, even for trials with encouraging findings, we may not fully comprehend how a particular herbal remedy functions [8]. Some of the treatments have been proven to reduce urine calcium excretion and increase urinary excretion of citrate, both of which affect urinary supersaturation. Herbs impede crystal nucleation, development, and aggregation, which prevents the embryonic stone from growing in size and from being retained within the confined renal tubules. Herbal remedies boost urinary output, encouraging urine flow through renal tubules and the clearance of the developing stone before it is too large to move and obstructs the tubular lumens. They might prevent the kidneys from producing reactive oxygen species, which are known to encourage crystal attachment and their retention in the kidneys by damaging the renal epithelium [9].

3. Anti-nephrolithiatic activity of bioactive compounds

3.1 Flavonoids

Flavonols, flavones, catechins, anthocyanidins, isoflavones, dihydroflavones, and chalcones can be produced from the thousands of plant chemicals known as flavonoids. Vegetables, fruits, nuts, spices, herbs, red wine, tea, and other foods and beverages also contain varying levels of these chemicals. One of the major classes of polyphenols is flavonoids, which have a wide range of pharmacological functions and have antioxidant effects [10]. Several flavonoids have shown renal protective properties against various nephrotoxic agents that often cause acute kidney injury (AKI) or chronic kidney disease (CKD), such as gentamycin, alcohol, nicotine, lead, or cadmium. Hemodialysis patients observed vasculoprotective benefits of cocoa flavanols in humans [11].

Many flavonoids such as quercitin, hyperoside, rutin, diosmin, and apigenin have been investigated for their probable potential to inhibit the formation of kidney stones. **Table 1** summarizes the main findings regarding the anti-nephrolithiatic activity of flavonoids [12–16].

3.2 Terpenoids

Naturally occurring pentacyclic triterpenes of plant origin can have a wide range of pharmacological effects. Lupeol and botulin(pentacyclic triterpenes) were similarly effective in reducing tissue damage brought on by crystal-induced renal peroxidative alterations as evaluated by malondialdehyde. The two substances may work by inhibiting calcium oxalate crystal aggregation and boosting the body's defensive mechanisms to provide protection against oxalate-induced toxic symptoms and free radical generation [17]. Moreover, childhood nephrolithiasis or urolithiasis has benefited significantly from the use of essential oil preparations of terpenic, which contain pinene (31%), camphene (15%), borneol (10%), anethol (4%), fenchone (4%), and cineol (3%). The majority of essential oil preparations are sold in the Middle East under the brand name Urinex (Pharco Co.) [18].

Compounds	Study type	Results	References
Quercetin	*In vivo*	Reduced damage due to hyperoxaluria. Reduced oxalate stone formation	[12]
Quercetin and hyperoside	*In vivo*	Reduced the number of crystal deposits Increased superoxide dismutase and catalase levels	[13]
Rutin	*In vivo*	Decreased calcium and oxalate in the urine Less tissue damage and fewer number of calcium oxalate deposits in kidney of animal	[14]
Diosmin	*In vivo*	The average volume of calcium oxalate in the nephrolithiasis+diosmin rats was -63% lower than in the rats with untreated nephrolithiasis..	[15]
Apigenin	*In vivo*	Reduced calcium levels in kidneys Enhanced renal function	[16]

Table 1.
Anti-nephrolithiatic activity of flavonoids.

3.3 Furanocoumarin

The impact of two furanochromes (khellin and visnagin) on ethylene-glycol-induced hyperoxaluria in rats was only discussed in one study elaborated by Vanachayangkul et al. [19]. In this work, khellin and visnagin effectively reduced the incidence of calcium oxalate (CaOx) crystal deposition in rats with nephrolithiasis at doses of 5 and 10 mg/kg/day. The authors of this study hypothesized that khellin and visnagin interfere with calcium blocking activity rather than citrate reabsorption, despite the fact that these two substances did not influence urine parameters (pH, citrate, calcium, and oxalate) in this investigation [19].

3.4 Phenolic acids

The potent pharmacological effects of phenolic acids include antioxidant, antibacterial, anticancer, antiviral, anti-inflammatory, antimutagenic, antirheumatic, antipyretic, antiseptic, anthelmintic, neuroprotective, and hepatoprotective properties [20].

Many phenolic acids such as ferulic acid, gallic acid, caffiec, and rosmarinic acid have been investigated for their probable ability to inhibit the formation of kidney stones. **Table 2** summarizes the main findings regarding the anti-nephrolithiatic activity of phenolic acids [21–24].

3.5 Tannins

Green tea contains a polyphenolic hydrolyzable tannin called gallotannin. At non-toxic concentrations, gallotannin dramatically reduced the development of CaOx monohydrate crystals and their attachment to MDCK I kidney epithelial cells. Additionally, gallotannin decreased the amount of reactive oxygen species (ROS) and malondialdehyde (MDA) produced by human primary renal epithelial cells and increased the activity of the antioxidant enzyme superoxide dismutase (SOD) in response to oxalate [25]. Catechin has proven successful in inhibiting renal papillary calcification and the growth of CaOx monohydrate papillary calculi, which may be related to its stimulation of SOD activity [26].

3.6 Saponins

The saponin-rich fraction made from the fruits of S. xanthocarpum prevented the nucleation and aggregation of calcium oxalate crystals in artificial urine solution in

Compounds	Study type	Results	References
Ferulic acid	*In vivo*	Inhibition of renal stone formation and oxidative stress. Increased lipid peroxidation	[21]
Caffeic acid	*In vivo*	Regulation of the changed biochemical parameters Reduction of calcium oxalate deposits.	[22]
Gallic acid	*In vivo*	Inhibition approximately 44-57% of the total calcium oxalate crystals formation,	[23]
Rosmarinic acid	*In vivo*	Decreased tubular dilatation, Bowman's capsule enlargement, degradation of the tubular epithelium, and localized glomerular necrosis.	[24]

Table 2.
Anti-nephrolithiatic activity of phenolic acids.

vitro, and it inhibited the pathological changes brought on by lithogenic treatment, such as polyuria, damage to renal function, oxidative stress, and crystalluria in rats with urolithiasis caused by EG [27].

3.7 Alkaloids

Evidence indicates that alkaloids can enhance urine production and Na^+ and K^+ excretion in a manner similar to that of a typical diuretic (hydrochlorothiazide). Additionally, it has been demonstrated that berberine therapy lowers the Ca^{2+} level of urine. Due to the excess calcium being the main requirement for crystal precipitation and one of the key risk factors for stone production, this has a lot of significance to urinary supersaturation [28].

4. The mechanistic insight of polyphenols in oxalate nephrolithiasis

4.1 Antioxidant

Due to the presence of flavonoids and vitamins, some plant extracts suggested to prevent nephrolithiasis, such as the FHE employed in this study, have a strong antioxidant potential. By preventing lipid peroxidation and papillary tip epithelium damage caused by hyperoxaluria, these substances may prevent the formation of calcium oxalate crystals in the kidney. This in turn may prevent heterogeneous calcium oxalate crystal nucleation on damaged cells or cellular debris, which leads to the development of kidney stones [24].

4.2 Diuretic

It has been frequently observed that polyphenols have diuretic properties. Traditional diuretics include extracts from the fruits of *Opuntia ficus indica*, *C. sinensis*, and *Hibiscus sabdariffa*. By flushing out the salt deposits, the diuretic action increases the amount of fluid going through the kidneys. Therefore, an increase in urine volume reduces salt saturation and prevents the crystals from precipitating at physiological pH [29].

4.3 Conclusions and perceptions

This chapter reveals the results obtained from the available literature about the bioactive components of medicinal plants such as flavonoids, terpenoids, tannins, saponins, etc. The majority of this research was exploratory, conducted on animals, and is insufficient for the creation of medicinal products. To evaluate the effectiveness and toxicity of these plants, extensive preclinical and clinical investigations are still needed. Future research on clinical applications may therefore be a profitable way to confirm the clinical utility of these medications.

Conflict of interest

"The authors declare no conflict of interest."

Author details

Farah Al-Mamoori[1*] and Talal Aburjai[2]

1 Faculty of Pharmacy, Department of Pharmaceutical Sciences, Zarqa University, Zarqa, Jordan

2 Faculty of Pharmacy, Department of Pharmaceutical Sciences, University of Jordan, Amman, Jordan

*Address all correspondence to: fmamoori@zu.edu.jo

References

[1] Romero V, Akpinar H, Assimos DG. Kidney stones: A global picture of prevalence, incidence, and associated risk factors. Reviews in Urology. 2010;**12**(2-3):e86

[2] Aldaher HS, Kadhim SZ, Al-Roub NM, Alsadi AH, Salam DA, Tillo EA. Evaluating the understanding about kidney stones among adults in the United Arab Emirates. Journal of Taibah University Medical Sciences. 2021;**16**(5):788-793. DOI: 10.1016/j.jtumed.2021.04.005

[3] Shirani M, Arjaki D, Kheiri S, Bijad E, Mohammadi S, Lorigooini Z. An in vitro screening potential traditional medicinal plants for nephrolithiasis. Clinical Phytoscience. 2020;**6**(1):1-8

[4] Akram M, Idrees M. Progress and prospects in the management of kidney stones and developments in phyto-therapeutic modalities. International Journal of Immunopathology and Pharmacology. 2019;**2019**:33. DOI: 10.1177/2058738419848220

[5] Sansores-España D, Pech-Aguilar AG, Cua-Pech KG, Medina-Vera I, Guevara-Cruz M, Gutiérrez-Solis AL, et al. Plants used in Mexican traditional medicine for the Management of Urolithiasis: A review of preclinical evidence, bioactive compounds, and molecular mechanisms. Molecules. 2022;**27**(6):2008. DOI: 10.3390/molecules27062008

[6] Khan SR. Reactive oxygen species, inflammation and calcium oxalate nephrolithiasis. Translational Andrology and Urology. 2014;**3**(3):256

[7] Kant R, Singh TG, Singh S. Mechanistic approach to herbal formulations used for urolithiasis treatment. Obesity Medicine. 2020;**19**:100266. DOI: 10.1016/j.obmed.2020.100266

[8] Grases F, Prieto RM, Gomila I, Sanchis P, Costa-Bauzá A. Phytotherapy and renal stones: The role of antioxidants. A pilot study in Wistar rats. Urological Research. 2009;**37**(1):35-40. DOI: 10.1007/s00240-008-0165-1

[9] Khan A, Khan SR. Clinical studies of medicinal plants for their antiurolithic effects: A systematic review. https://doi.org/10.21037/lcm-21-51

[10] Middleton E, Kandaswami C, Theoharides TC. The effects of plant flavonoids on mammalian cells: Implications for inflammation, heart disease, and cancer. Pharmacological Reviews. 2000;**52**(4):673-751

[11] Vargas F, Romecín P, García-Guillén AI, Wangesteen R, Vargas-Tendero P, Paredes MD, et al. Flavonoids in kidney health and disease. Frontiers in Physiology. 2018;**24**:394. DOI: 10.3389/fphys.2018.00394

[12] Guzel A, Yunusoglu S, Calapoglu M, Candan IA, Onaran I, Oncu M, et al. Protective effects of quercetin on oxidative stress-induced tubular epithelial damage in the experimental rat hyperoxaluria model. Medicina. 2021;**57**(6):566. DOI: 10.3390/medicina57060566

[13] Zhu W, Xu YF, Feng Y, Peng B, Che JP, Liu M, et al. Prophylactic effects of quercetin and hyperoside in a calcium oxalate stone forming rat model. Urolithiasis. 2014;**42**(6):519-526

[14] Ghodasara J, Pawar A, Deshmukh C, Kuchekar B. Inhibitory effect of rutin

and curcumin on experimentally-induced calcium oxalate urolithiasis in rats. Pharmacognosy. Research. 2010;**2**(6):388

[15] Noorafshan A, Karbalay-Doust S, Karimi F. Diosmin reduces calcium oxalate deposition and tissue degeneration in nephrolithiasis in rats: A stereological study. Korean Journal of Urology. 2013;**54**(4):252-257

[16] Stiani SN, Syahidah FM, Fikriani H, Subarnas A, Rusdiana T. Anticalculi activity of apigenin and celery (Apium Graveolens L.) extract in rats induced by ethylene glycol-ammonium chloride. The Journal of Pharmacy and Bioallied Sciences. 2019;**11**:S556-S561

[17] Malini MM, Lenin M, Varalakshmi P. Protective effect of triterpenes on calcium oxalate crystal-induced peroxidative changes in experimental urolithiasis. Pharmacological Research. 2000;**41**(4):413-418

[18] Al-Mosawi AJ. The treatment of childhood progressive bilateral multiple renal stone disease: A role of essential oil terpenes. Archive of Urological Research. 2020;**4**(1):007-009

[19] Vanachayangkul P, Chow N, Khan SR, Butterweck V. Prevention of renal crystal deposition by an extract of Ammi visnaga L. and its constituents khellin and visnagin in hyperoxaluric rats. Urological Research. 2011;**39**(3):189-195

[20] Heleno SA, Martins A, Queiroz MJRP, Ferreira ICFR. Bioactivity of phenolic acids: Metabolites versus parent compounds: A review. Food Chemistry. 2015;**173**:501-513

[21] Zhao B, Su B, Zhang H, Liu W, Du Q, Li Y. Antiurolithiatic effect of ferulic acid on ethylene glycolinduced renal calculus in experimental rats. Tropical Journal of Pharmaceutical Research. 2019;**18**(1):109-115

[22] Yasir F, Wahab AT, Choudhary MI. Protective effect of dietary polyphenol caffeic acid on ethylene glycol-induced kidney stones in rats. Urolithiasis. 2018;**46**(2):157-166

[23] Cechinel-Zanchett CC, Mariano LB, Schlickmann F, Cechinel-Filho V, de Souza P. In vitro effects of two bioactive compounds, gallic acid and methyl gallate, on urolithiasis. Actas Urológicas Españolas (English Edition). 2021;**45**(9):604-608. DOI: 10.1016/j.acuro.2020.09.016

[24] Öztürk H, Öztürk H, Terzi EH, Özgen U, Duran A. Protective effects of rosmarinic acid against renal ischaemia/reperfusion injury in rats. Journal of the Pakistan Medical Association. 2014;**64**(3):260-265

[25] Lee HJ, Jeong SJ, Park MN, Linnes M, Han HJ, Kim JH, et al. Gallotannin suppresses calcium oxalate crystal binding and oxalate-induced oxidative stress in renal epithelial cells. Biological and Pharmaceutical Bulletin. 2012;**35**(4):539-544

[26] Patel P, Patel M, Saralai M, Gandhi T. Antiurolithiatic effects of Solanum xanthocarpum fruit extract on ethylene-glycol-induced nephrolithiasis in rats. Journal of Young Pharmacists. 2012;**4**:164-170

[27] Bashir S, Gilani AH, Siddiqui AA, Pervez S, Khan SR, Sarfaraz NJ, et al. Berberis vulgaris root bark extract prevents hyperoxaluria induced urolithiasis in rats. Phytotherapy Research. 2010;**24**:1250-1255. DOI: 10.1002/ptr.3196

[28] Grases F, Costa-Bauzá A, Prieto RM, Conte A, Servera A. Renal papillary

calcification and the development of calcium oxalate monohydrate papillary renal calculi: A case series study. BMC Urology. 2013;**13**(1):1-7

[29] Ahmed S, Hasan MM, Khan H, Mahmood ZA, Patel S. The mechanistic insight of polyphenols in calcium oxalate urolithiasis mitigation. Biomedicine & Pharmacotherapy. 2018;**106**:1292-1299

Section 2

Stone Prevention

Chapter 5

Stone Prevention: Dietary Factors, Current Evidence, and Metabolic Workup

Wajahat Aziz, Ahmad Bashir and Mohammad Hammad Ather

Abstract

Urolithiasis is a highly recurrent disease. The incidence of urolithiasis is on the rise. Although stone prevention is highly desirable, there is significant controversy and lack of quality evidence to suggest a standard approach to prevention. In the current chapter, we have looked at the contemporary evidence, lack of long-term compliance, and various dietary and pharmacological treatment options for prevention of recurrent stone disease.

Keywords: prevention, metaphylaxis, translational research, dietary factors, urolithiasis

1. Introduction

Urolithiasis is an endemic condition in certain parts of the world, particularly where weather is dry and hot. However, current data suggest that it is now increasingly identified in high income countries and its prevalence is independent of the weather conditions. Genetic and dietary influences are two important predispositions. Urolithiasis is now considered as a systemic disorder. The exact etiology is still elusive, however, there is a complex and intricate interplay of genetic and dietary factory. The epigenetics play provides an important link between environment and genetics. Urolithiasis is not only highly prevalent but has a very high recurrence risk. This chapter looks at the various preventive strategies, the contemporary evidence in support and influence of diet on urolithiasis prevention.

2. Why stone prevention is important?

An episode of ureteric colic or urosepsis secondary to urinary stones is an alarming experience for a patient. In many cases, stones may require medical or invasive endourological procedures to remove them with its attendant cost and morbidity. The estimated cost of urolithiasis management is likely to be ~$4.1 billion by 2030 in United States alone [1]. Additionally, recurrent kidney stones can lead to long-term complications and continue to be a significant cause of end stage renal disease in the developing world [2].

3. Patients with high risk of stone recurrence

The risk of recurrence after the first stone episode may be as high as 90% in 5 years. However, this risk is quite variable and depends upon several patient and stone-related factors. A subset of patients is identifiable for which the risk of recurrence is much higher [3]. These patients should be specifically directed for metabolic workup and implementation of stone prevention strategies.

3.1 Patient factors

Age at first stone episode, number of previous episodes, time since last stone episode, family history, male gender, and body mass index are important predictors of stone recurrence.

3.2 Some other factors

Uric acid, struvite, and brushite stones are more likely to recur as compared to calcium oxalate stones [4]. Singh and colleagues [5] noted that symptomatic recurrence at 10 years was approximately 50% for brushite, struvite, and uric acid but approximately 30% for calcium oxalate and hydroxyapatite stones ($P < .001$). Patients with cystine stones can have an episode of stone requiring intervention almost every year or even more frequently [6]. Moreover, patients with a greater number and size of stones at first presentation and those with bilateral stones are more likely to experience recurrence of the disorder.

3.3 Specific medical conditions

Rarely during basic workup is a specific medical condition identifiable which increases the risk of stone recurrence such as gout, renal tubular acidosis, obesity, diabetes, cystinuria, recurrent UTI, or hyperparathyroidism [7, 8].

Dietary and social habits such as dehydration, a high intake of sodium, and animal protein all increase the risk of stone recurrence [9].

4. Difficulties in developing stone prevention strategies

Multiple factors have traditionally shifted the focus of research away from stone prevention. Firstly, the safety and efficacy of endoscopic stone removal have increased exponentially over the last few decades. This has shifted the focus to early diagnosis and intervention for stones, whereas workup to determine a specific cause of stones does not always provide useful answers. The mainstay of workup namely 24-hour urinalysis for identifying metabolic factors is cumbersome and usually not a true representative of patient's day-to-day life [10]. Lastly, even if a specific metabolic abnormality is identified, it may not be amenable to a specific treatment [11].

Preventing stone recurrence involves identifying the underlying causes of the stones and implementing strategies to address those causes. Developing stone prevention strategies is challenging due to several factors, including the following:

4.1 Complexity of stone formation

Kidney stone formation is a complex process that involves several factors, including genetics, diet, and environmental factors. The simple pathogenesis of solutes increasing the supersaturation of urine with respect to one of the stone constituents does not completely account for all these factors, whereas prevention strategies have mostly focused on either increasing the quantity of the solvent (i.e., water) or reducing that of the solutes (e.g., calcium, sodium, and oxalate) [12].

4.2 Limited understanding of dietary factors

Diet plays an important role in the development of kidney stones, but there is still limited understanding and lack of evidence for the role of specific dietary factors other than water intake and their contribution to stone formation.

4.3 Patient adherence

Stone prevention strategies often require significant lifestyle changes, such as increased fluid intake and dietary modifications. However, patient adherence to these changes can be challenging, which can limit the effectiveness of prevention strategies.

4.4 Limited access to health care

Stone prevention strategies may require access to specialized healthcare services, such as urology and nephrology. However, limited access to these services in some areas can make it difficult for patients to receive appropriate care and follow-up [13].

4.5 Cost

Developing effective stone prevention strategies may require significant investment in research, education, and healthcare services. The cost of these efforts can be a barrier to the development and implementation of effective prevention strategies.

5. Empiric therapy

The fact that stones are the outcome of multiple genetic, dietary, and environmental causes along with difficulties in identifying specific factors and targeting them for stone prevention has shifted focus toward a more generic empiric therapy [14]. This can be applied to all patients presenting with renal stones without subjecting them to the cost and burden of a detailed workup. However, it cannot be overemphasized that some of the patients who are at greater risk of recurrence, as mentioned above, or have a stone type other than calcium and uric acid stones, should be identified for targeted therapy.

5.1 Fluid intake

A Cochrane review published in 2019 evaluated the effectiveness of increasing water intake as a prevention strategy for kidney stones. The review analyzed three randomized controlled trials with a total of 255 participants that compared increased water intake to standard fluid intake. The review found that increasing water intake reduced the risk of kidney stone formation by 50%. The effect was most significant for individuals with a history of calcium oxalate stones. This provides strong evidence to support the importance of adequate water intake as a key prevention strategy for all kidney stones specially calcium oxalate stones.

Recent studies have also suggested that the timing and distribution of water intake throughout the day, known as circadian water intake, may also play a role in the prevention of urolithiasis [15]. Drinking water at regular intervals throughout the day can help to maintain adequate hydration levels and reduce the risk of stone formation by keeping the concentration of stone-forming substances like calcium and oxalate below their formation product [16].

5.2 Weight loss

Reducing weight can play a significant role in preventing renal stones, especially if the stones are caused by metabolic syndrome. Obesity is associated with insulin resistance, which can lead to increased urinary excretion of oxalate and calcium [17]. Moreover, insulin resistance can lead to metabolic acidosis, which lowers urinary pH, thereby promoting uric acid stone formation [18]. Losing weight can improve insulin sensitivity, thereby reducing the urinary excretion of oxalate and the risk of kidney stone formation [19].

5.3 Generic dietary manipulations

These include limiting sodium and animal protein intake besides maintaining a diet rich in fruits and fibers. A high intake of sodium can increase calcium excretion in the urine, thereby promoting stone formation. Limiting sodium intake to less than 2300 milligrams per day as per American Heart Association Guidelines, i.e., not more than 3–5 g of salt has been found to lower the risk of renal stones as well [20].

Several studies have linked a high intake of animal protein to an increased risk of kidney stones [21–23]. However, it is important to note that not all animal proteins are equally problematic when it comes to kidney stone risk. Fish and dairy products, for example, have been shown to have a protective effect against kidney stones (references required). This may be due to the high magnesium and citrate content of these foods, which can help prevent the formation of kidney stones. A systematic review of 14 prospective cohort studies studying the effect of total protein and protein sources showed that each 5% increase in total protein intake was associated with a 10% increase in kidney stone risk [22].

A balanced diet that includes plenty of fruits and vegetables can help reduce the risk of kidney stones. This may be partially due to a reduction in animal proteins and salts in such a diet. However, diets high in citrus fruits and low-fat dairy products have been shown specifically to prevent stone formation [24].

5.4 Empiric medications

These include prescription for potassium citrate, allopurinol, and thiazides without specifically analyzing a 24-hour urine. A comparison of empiric medications based upon clinical assessment alone with targeted therapy based upon 24-hour urine analysis showed that targeted therapy is not better than empiric therapy in reducing the risk of stone recurrence [25]. However, a similar comparison for high-risk groups including children indicated that targeted therapy is more likely to reduce stone recurrence in high-risk groups [26]. Therefore, a stratified approach of using empiric therapy for low-risk groups and targeted therapy for those with high risk of recurrence is appropriate.

6. Targeted therapy

Several advances in the field of precision medicine have improved our ability to identify and target specific risk factors for kidney stone formation. For example, genetic testing can identify inherited mutations that increase the risk of certain types of stones, while spot metabolic testing can measure urine and blood levels of key substances involved in stone formation avoiding the cumbersome 24-hour urine collection.

Using this information, clinicians can address the specific factors contributing to a patient's stone formation. This may include lifestyle modifications, dietary changes, and medications such as thiazide diuretics, citrates, and allopurinol.

6.1 Thiazide diuretics

Generally, a low dose of a thiazide diuretic, such as hydrochlorothiazide 12.5–25 mg/day is best suited for patients with documented hypercalciuria. By inhibiting the Na^+/Cl^- co-transporter, thiazide diuretics reduce sodium reabsorption in the distal convoluted tubule, thereby increasing calcium reabsorption. A meta-analysis of 8 RCTs (what does this mean?) involving 571 patients showed that thiazide diuretics almost halved the risk of stone recurrence but at the expense of side effects leading to poor patient compliance [27]. This is one of the main reasons that thiazide diuretics are less commonly used for this indication.

6.2 Citrate

Citrate is commonly used for the prevention of kidney stones, particularly those composed of calcium oxalate or calcium phosphate. Citrate can be given in the form of potassium citrate or potassium citrate. Citrate acts by binding to calcium in the urine, which reduces the amount of calcium available to form stones. Citrate also raises the pH of the urine, which makes it less favorable for stone formation. Studies have shown that citrate therapy is effective in reducing the risk of recurrent kidney stones. A Cochrane review of seven trials involving 477 patients showed that citrate therapy reduced the risk of recurrent stones by 75%. Citrate therapy was also associated with a reduction in stone burden and fewer surgical interventions [28].

6.3 Xanthine oxidase inhibitors

By inhibiting xanthine oxidase, allopurinol increases the levels of hypoxanthine and xanthine, which are more soluble than uric acid and are more readily excreted in the urine. While allopurinol is an effective medication for the prevention of uric acid stones, there are practical problems that limit its long-term use including adherence and cost. In one study, patients who were non-adherent to medication, were more likely to require surgical treatment for stone recurrence [29]. Febuxostat in another xanthine oxidase inhibitor is more effective in reducing uric acid levels both in blood and urine. However, this does not necessarily translate into a greater clinical effectiveness in preventing renal stones [30].

7. From lab to the clinic in stone research

Translation research in urolithiasis is essentially a process of covering an observation made in the laboratory, clinic, or community into an intervention that provides meaningful and applicable results. In the area of urolithiasis, it has impacted two major domains of management, i.e., firstly, the active management which is treatment of the stone itself and, secondly, the prevention of recurrence which is a major issue. Indeed, there has been significant progress in the first domain which is active management. Open stone surgery has been completely replaced by endourology even in the developing world [31]. Even the most complex kidney stones can be treated by minimally invasive surgery.

Kidney stone disease is a systemic disorder. The overall prevalence in the general population is increasing. In the USA, datum indicates that 1 in 11 persons have a kidney stone. This is almost equivalent to the prevalence of diabetes. Besides the high incidence of *de novo* stones, there is a high recurrence rate which together not only have a cost implication but also a significant impact on the overall health of patients. Stone prevention is therefore important, and measures are likely to not only decrease the recurrence but may have beneficial effect on other heath related matters. Shadman and Bastani [32] noted that urolithiasis is associated with chronic kidney disease, hematologic cancers, various endocrine disorders and metabolic syndrome, type 2 DM, autoimmune diseases, inflammatory bowel diseases, bone loss and fractures, hypertension, and coronary heart diseases and most recently ischemic strokes.

The first step in stone prevention is to identify the cause in an individual patient. Ferraro et al. [33] shared interesting datum concerning the practice patterns in various European and non-European centers. In this survey, the authors noted that a basic blood workup is performed in most patients and nutritional advice and stone composition analysis are carried out in a significant proportion. However, the 24-hour urinary parameters are not assessed in every patient. About half of the patients have only 7 out of 16 parameters assessed. So, the question is that when should it be done and in whom? In the review by Coninck, Keller and Traxer [34], they advised that medical and lifestyle history, physical examination, basic urine and blood workup, radiological examination, and stone analysis should be performed in all patients. Detailed 24-hour urine analysis is indicated in patients who are at high risk of recurrent stone disease. In a review written by us about five years ago, we also advocated the use of a tailored metabolic workup for urolithiasis which should be performed on selective individuals [35].

DOI: http://dx.doi.org/10.5772/intechopen.111809

Currently we lack quality evidence regarding stone prevention strategies. In a meta-analysis from the Cochrane database, it is noted that there no RCT (what does this mean?) on the role of increased water intake for the primary prevention of urinary stones. However, for secondary stone prevention, increasing urinary output to achieve a two-liter volume is suggested. The "PUSH trial" [36] is an interesting proposal published in the American Journal of Kidney Diseases for the prevention of urinary stone with hydration. One of the fundamental problems with advice related to lifestyle is the lack of compliance. The proposed trial is set to study in a randomized trial of a multicomponent behavioral intervention program to increase and maintain a high fluid intake. Participants are randomly assigned (1:1 ratio) to the intervention or control arm. The proposed sample size is 1642 subjects.

In pediatric urolithiasis, there is very little controversy about the role of metabolic analysis to identify the cause of the stone and treating the patient to prevent long-term morbidity and stone recurrence. Compliance and tolerating medications are a greater issue. In a recent Cochrane database systematic review authors noted that oral potassium citrate supplementation may reduce recurrent calcium stone formation in children following lithotripsy. However, the majority of children poorly tolerate potassium citrate [37].

Besides the indication for metabolic workup, the main controversy is the extent of the workup. It is important to assess minerals forming stones like calcium, oxalate, uric acid, phosphate, etc. One also needs to assess what prevents stones such as citrate and stone promoters such as sodium, since hypernatriuria leads to hypercalciuria. Extremes of urinary pH may result in the either uric acid or magnesium ammonium phosphate and calcium phosphate stones. Potassium and creatinine estimations are indicators of adequacy of the specimen and compliance with treatment. Urine microscopy indicates the presence of bacteria. Red cells and white cells indicate that there is a likelihood of not only mechanical irritation secondary to stone but also urine tract infection. The presence of crystals, like those typical of cystine, is indicative of cystinuria. The coffin-lid crystals of magnesium ammonium phosphate and the double tetrahedrons of calcium oxalate dihydrate are also indicative of these respective types of stones. Kidney stone disease is associated with so many other conditions; for example, recurrent calcium oxalate urolithiasis is associated with osteoporosis, and it is not old-age osteoporosis as it is seen in male patients aged 35 years and female patients aged only 38 years. Dexascan can identify patients who have osteoporosis versus osteopenia and normal density [38]. Stone analysis to identify the mineral contents and composition is of utmost importance.

Interpretation of the findings is the next logical step. Following analysis, stones are broadly classified into calcium-containing or non-calcium containing. In the case of calcium-containing stones, you need to measure urinary calcium excretion. For normocalciuric patients, however, one needs to look for other risk factors such as hyperuricosuria, hyperoxaluria, and hypocitraturia. For hypercalciuric patients, serum calcium and PTH levels should be performed, and the patients treated appropriately. Non-calcium stones such as uric acid, cystine or infection-related stones should be treated accordingly [39].

In an interesting study, the authors noted that the consumption of carbonated drinks (which are high in phosphoric acid) in the presence of *Proteus mirabil*is infection can cause struvite stones [40]. Residual stone becomes the nidus for stone formation. In this study by Sorensen et al. [41], the authors concluded that removal of secondary small stones at the time of primary stone removal significantly decreases the chances of relapse without increasing surgery-related complications.

Most of the patients have calcium oxalate stones, without any metabolic disorder.

8. Stone prevention; dietary components

Before embarking on to a topic as vast as the role of diet in kidney stone prevention, it is imperative to first revisit briefly some of the well-known basics about stone formation itself. Kidney stones are aggregates composed of varying amounts of crystalloid substances. While theories explaining stone formation remain incomplete at best, there is an undeniable underlying role of supersaturation of urine in stone formation. Supersaturation of urine, in turn, is dependent on three major determinants, namely solute content, solvent volume, and the pH of urine, and consequently, any factor that were to alter any of these determinants would have an eventual effect on stone formation to some degree [42]. It is also useful to be familiar with certain concepts. The first of these is solubility product, at which point the solvent has reached its limit of solute content, and a further increase in ionic content beyond this point can potentially result in crystal nucleation [43]. The reason why this usually does not occur is the basis of the second concept, namely the presence of certain urinary constituents referred to as "inhibitors", which, as their name implies, oppose the formation of stones. As with the ionic concentration, alteration of the concentration of inhibitors would likewise have an eventual effect on stone formation. While in theory ions can still aggregate at their solubility product, the likelihood of doing so increases many-fold once they attain higher concentrations, a phenomenon referred to as the formation product [44] of the salt or acid concerned. It is postulated that concentrations beyond this point are unstable and can spontaneously initiate the process of crystal formation that may lead to stones. Lastly, it is important to be aware of different ions present in urine. To recall, the most important ions for causing stones include calcium, oxalate, phosphate, uric acid, and sodium [45], while the protective ions (inhibitors) mainly include citrate, magnesium, and sulphate. Rogers et al. [46] noted that increasing urinary sulfate could theoretically reduce calcium oxalate and calcium phosphate stone risk. The detailed role of each in stone formation is beyond the scope of this chapter. With this information, let us now proceed to the role of diet in stone formation.

Dietary factors can be approached in a variety of ways. The author's preference is to divide dietary items into food items and beverage items and the resultant impact of each on stone formation. It is pertinent to remember that renal stones have been increasingly linked to obesity and arterial hypertension, and hence, diet that predisposes to these latter conditions can reasonably be associated to have an indirect relationship with stone formation.

The paucity of randomized trials on diet entails that most information on the subject is derived from cohort studies.

8.1 Beverages

The effect of an increased fluid intake is beneficial with respect to stone formation, mainly because of increased dilution of the ionic solutes, decreased supersaturation, and the resultant prevention of crystal nucleation. This inverse relationship has been demonstrated in several studies [47, 48]. However, as pointed out before, fluids that cause changes in urinary pH or ion-rich fluids can have varying effects. Most experts agree that the 24-hour fluid intake for stone prevention should be approximately 2.5 to 3 liters and that this intake be circadian rather than bolus-like at varied intervals [49]. Simultaneously, the target urine volume should be approximately 2 to 2.5 liters (higher for certain pathological conditions) [50]. While the effects of beverage-induced reduced incidence of stone formation are attributable mainly to increased solubility of ions in urine, certain beverages including alcohol, coffee, and tea have an additional mechanism of stone prevention through promotion of diuresis with or without natriuresis. The only exception is soda, which has inconsistently been shown to increase the risk of stone formation, likely owing to its effect on the increased excretion of calcium, oxalate, and uric acid. The effect of fruit juices is mainly determined by the presence of citrate or bicarbonate and can work both ways [51]. Citric juices including lemon, orange, and grapefruit provide a high load of citrate and in theory can be a good alternate to pharmacotherapy [52]. However, fruit juices are also a source of sugar and oxalate, and hence, consumption should be limited to one glass per day, diluted in water.

8.2 Diet

One way to look at dietary factors is to employ a balanced-diet approach and avoiding excess of any food groups. However, it is helpful to elucidate the contribution of different food items to urinary ions, especially in situations where an individual is prone to forming a certain type of stone owing to an underlying abnormality.

Meat intake is significantly associated with risk of stone formation (reference!). This relationship has been consistently observed in observational studies and is attributed to higher levels of calcium, uric acid and possibly oxalate in urine, lower levels of citrate, and a lower urinary pH favoring the formation of both calcium and uric acid stones. There have been attempts to differentiate between red meat, processed meat, and poultry, and while the quality of the evidence remains low, a significant association was demonstrable with red meat while mixed results were found with poultry and fish, varying from null to a significant association. The consensus is to limit animal protein intake to 1 gram per kilogram per day [53] .

Fruits have a protective effect against stone formation owing to their citrate and potassium content. Dietary citrate is absorbed in the gastrointestinal tract and metabolized to bicarbonate, which may then increase urine pH and citrate excretion [54]. A similar effect on urine has been noted with potassium supplements [55].

Vegetables have been shown to exert the same effect as fruits, which seems to be linked to both the mechanisms linked above, or simply because a diet that is rich in vegetables is more likely to be lower in meat content. The main concern, however, is the presence of oxalate in certain vegetables such as spinach, beetroot, soya beans, and okra, all of which have the potential to cause mild hyperoxaluria with resultant stone formation. A reasonable advice is to restrict the aforementioned vegetables, however they can other leafy vegetables like cabbage, green peas, and turnip that have a lower oxalate content [56, 57].

While they are not food items in their own accord, the roles of calcium and sodium have also been well studied. Calcium complexes with oxalate in the gut to prevent its reabsorption and resultant excretion in urine. Thus, calcium intake must not be reduced, especially in people known to have hyperoxaluria, and should adhere to the recommended daily allowance of 1000–1200 mg/day [58]. Higher intake can potentially result in hypercalciuria. Sodium has been shown to be a promoter of hypercalciuria with a simultaneous decrease in citrate. While the intake of sodium should not exceed 3–5 grams per day, a reasonable rule of thumb is to avoid adding salt to food at the table [28].

While it is useful to know what the effect of a certain nutrient is, it might be difficult to individualize these nutrients in each meal. Hence, a wiser approach would be to target dietary patterns. One such program is the dietary approaches to stop hypertension (DASH) diet. A diet rich in fruits and vegetables, and low in saturated fat, is advised. It has been shown to have a beneficial effect on the urinary composition with higher levels of inhibitors and lower levels of supersaturates [59].

As pointed out earlier in the text, dietary prevention of stone disease is a vast topic, and all aspects concerning interactions at the ionic level are beyond the scope of this chapter. However, the data can be summarized quite conveniently for the sake of better patient understanding and compliance. Circadian fluid intake with neutral pH beverages to maintain a urine output volume of 2–2.5 liters is the cornerstone of preventive measures. Patients should be encouraged to maintain a balanced diet comprising a high intake of fruits, vegetables and fiber, a moderate intake of animal protein, and a low intake of salt, while avoiding excess of any particular food group.

While the role of dietary factors in the prevention of stones is vital, it is crucial to remember that stone disease has also been linked to higher calorie intake, higher body mass index, and cardiovascular disease. Therefore, dietary recommendations should be made into consideration of an overall healthier lifestyle including exercise. Furthermore, the majority of the conclusions are drawn from large cohort studies, and stronger randomized trials will likely be needed to confirm what is already known.

Author details

Wajahat Aziz[1], Ahmad Bashir[2] and Mohammad Hammad Ather[1]*

1 Aga Khan University, Karachi, Pakistan

2 Department of Surgery, Aga Khan University, Lahore, Pakistan

*Address all correspondence to: hammad.ather@aku.edu

References

[1] Bayne DB, Chi TL. Assessing cost-effectiveness of new technologies in stone management. Urologic Clinics. 2019;**46**(2):303-313

[2] Chuang TF, Hung HC, Li SF, Lee MW, Pai JY, Hung CT. Risk of chronic kidney disease in patients with kidney stones—A nationwide cohort study. BMC Nephrology. 2020;**21**:1-7

[3] Vaughan LE, Enders FT, Lieske JC, Pais VM, Rivera ME, Mehta RA, et al. Predictors of symptomatic kidney stone recurrence after the first and subsequent episodes. In: Mayo Clinic Proceedings. Vol. 94, No. 2. Elsevier Inc.; 2019. pp. 202-210

[4] Thongprayoon C, Krambeck AE, Rule AD. Determining the true burden of kidney stone disease. Nature Reviews Nephrology. 2020;**16**(12):736-746

[5] Singh P, Enders FT, Vaughan LE, Bergstrah EJ, Knoedler JJ, Krembeck AJ, et al. Stone composition among first-time symptomatic kidney stone formers in the community. Mayo Clinic Proceedings. 2015;**90**(10):1356-1365. DOI: 10.1016/j.mayocp.2015.07. 016 Epub 2015 Sep 6

[6] Piñero-Fernández JA, Vicente-Calderón C, Lorente-Sánchez MJ, et al. Phenotypic characterization of a pediatric cohort with cystinuria and usefulness of newborn screening. Berlin, Germany: Pediatric Nephrology; May 2023;**38**(5):1513-1521

[7] Taylor EN, Stampfer MJ, Curhan GC. Obesity, weight gain, and the risk of kidney stones. JAMA. 2005;**293**(4):455-462

[8] Taylor EN, Stampfer MJ, Curhan GC. Diabetes mellitus and the risk of nephrolithiasis. Kidney International. 2005;**68**(3):1230-1235

[9] Bargagli M, Tio MC, Waikar SS, Ferraro PM. Dietary oxalate intake and kidney outcomes. Nutrients. 2020;**12**(9):2673. DOI: 10.3390/nu12092673

[10] Parks JH, Goldfisher E, Asplin JR, Coe FL. A single 24-hour urine collection is inadequate for the medical evaluation of nephrolithiasis. The Journal of Urology. 2002;**167**(4):1607-1612

[11] Zisman AL. Effectiveness of treatment modalities on kidney stone recurrence. Clinical Journal of the American Society of Nephrology. 2017;**12**(10):1699-1708

[12] Colussi G, De Ferrari ME, Brunati C, Civati G. Medical prevention, and treatment of urinary stones. Journal of Nephrology. 2000;**13**(Suppl 3):S65-S70

[13] Scotland KB, Armas-Phan M, Dominique G, Bayne D. Social determinants of kidney stone disease: The impact of race, income and access on urolithiasis treatment and outcomes. Urology. 2022;**163**:190-195

[14] Goldfarb DS. Empiric therapy for kidney stones. Urolithiasis. 2019;**47**(1):107-113

[15] Yitgin Y, Asrak H, Tefik T. Role, importance and assessment of dietary habits in urolithiasis patient. World Journal of Urology. May 2023;**41**(5):1229-1233

[16] Ferraro PM, Baccaro R, Baroni S, D'Alessandri L, Carpenito C, Di Daniele N, et al. Effect of water

composition and timing of ingestion on urinary lithogenic profile in healthy volunteers: A randomized crossover trial. Journal of Nephrology. 2021;**34**:875-881

[17] Sáenz-Medina J, Jorge E, Corbacho C, Santos M, Sánchez A, Soblechero P, et al. Metabolic syndrome contributes to renal injury mediated by hyperoxaluria in a murine model of nephrolithiasis. Urolithiasis. 2018;**46**:179-186

[18] Fu Q, Xie L, Diao C, Aizezi X, Liu X, Liu C. The impacts of metabolic syndrome on the risk of severe urolithiasis. Urolithiasis. 2022;**50**(4):423-430

[19] Sasaki Y, Kohjimoto Y, Iba A, Matsumura N, Hara I. Weight loss intervention reduces the risk of kidney stone formation in a rat model of metabolic syndrome. International Journal of Urology. 2015;**22**(4):404-409

[20] Kiremit MC, Boyuk A, Petkova K. Fluid intake recommendations in urolithiasis and general advice to patients without metabolic risk factors. World Journal of Urology. May 2023;**41**(5):1251-1259

[21] Heilberg IP, Goldfarb DS. Optimum nutrition for kidney stone disease. Advances in Chronic Kidney Disease. 2013;**20**(2):165-174. DOI: 10.1053/j.ackd.2012.12.001

[22] Asoudeh F, Talebi S, Jayedi A, Marx W, Najafi MT, Mohammadi H. Associations of Total protein or animal protein intake and animal protein sources with risk of kidney stones: A systematic review and dose-response meta-analysis. Advances in Nutrition. 2022;**13**(3):821-832. DOI: 10.1093/advances/nmac013

[23] Shu X, Calvert JK, Cai H, Xiang YB, Li H, Zheng W, et al. Plant and animal protein intake and risk of incident kidney stones: Results from the Shanghai Men's and Women's health studies. The Journal of Urology. 2019;**202**(6):1217-1223

[24] Lin BB, Lin ME, Huang RH, Hong YK, Lin BL, He XJ. Dietary and lifestyle factors for primary prevention of nephrolithiasis: A systematic review and meta-analysis. BMC nephrology. 2020;**21**(1):1-3

[25] Hsi RS, Yan PL, Goldfarb DS, Egbuji A, Si Y, Shahinian V, et al. Comparison of selective versus empiric pharmacologic preventative therapy with kidney stone recurrence. Urology. 2021;**149**:81-88

[26] Hsi RS, Yan PL, Crivelli JJ, Goldfarb DS, Shahinian V, Hollingsworth JM. Comparison of selective vs empiric pharmacologic preventive therapy of kidney stone recurrence with high-risk features. Urology. 2022;**164**:74-79

[27] Li DF, Gao YL, Liu HC, Huang XC, Zhu RF, Zhu CT. Use of thiazide diuretics for the prevention of recurrent kidney calculi: A systematic review and meta-analysis. Journal of Translational Medicine. 2020;**18**:1-2

[28] Phillips R, Hanchanale VS, Myatt A, Somani B, Nabi G, Biyani CS. Citrate salts for preventing and treating calcium containing kidney stones in adults. Cochrane Database of Systematic Reviews. 6 Oct 2015;**2015**(10):CD010057

[29] Canales BK, Sharma N, Yuzhakov SV, Bozorgmehri S, Otto BJ, Bird VG. Long-term recurrence rates in uric acid stone formers with or without medical management. Urology. 2019 Sep;**1**(131):46-52

[30] Goldfarb DS, MacDonald PA, Gunawardhana L, Chefo S, McLean L. Randomized controlled trial of febuxostat versus allopurinol or placebo

in individuals with higher urinary uric acid excretion and calcium stones. Clinical Journal of the American Society of Nephrology. 2013;**8**(11):1960-1967

[31] El-Husseiny T, Buchholz N. The role of open stone surgery. Arab Journal of Urology. 2012;**10**(3):284-288

[32] Shadman A, Bastani B. Kidney calculi: Pathophysiology and as a systemic disorder. Iranian Journal of Kidney Diseases. 2017;**11**(3):180-191

[33] Ferraro PM, Unwin R, Bonny O, Gambaro G. Practice patterns of kidney stone management across European and non-European centers: An in-depth investigation from the European renal stone network (ERSN). Journal of Nephrology. 2021;**34**(4):1337-1346. DOI: 10.1007/s40620-020-00854-6 Epub 2020 Sep 12

[34] De Coninck V, Keller EX, Traxer O. Metabolic evaluation: Who, when and how often. Current Opinion in Urology. 2019;**29**(1):52-64. DOI: 10.1097/MOU.0000000000000562

[35] Ather MH, Sulaiman MN, Siddiqui I, Siddiqui T. Tailored metabolic workup for Urolithiasis - the debate continues. Journal of the College of Physicians and Surgeons–Pakistan. 2017;**27**(2):101-104

[36] Scales CD Jr, Desai AC, Harper JD, Lai HH, Maalouf NM, Reese PP, et al. Urinary stone disease research network. Prevention of urinary stones with hydration (PUSH): Design and rationale of a clinical trial. American Journal of Kidney Diseases. 2021;**77**(6):898-906. e1. DOI: 10.1053/j.ajkd.2020.09.016 Epub 2020 Nov 16

[37] Kern A, Grimsby G, Mayo H, Baker LA. Medical and dietary interventions for preventing recurrent urinary stones in children. Cochrane Database of Systematic Reviews. 2017;**11**(11):CD011252

[38] Tugcu V, Ozbek E, Aras B, Ozbay B, Islim F, Tasci AI. Bone mineral density measurement in patients with recurrent normocalciuric calcium stone disease. Urological Research. 2007;**35**(1):29-34. DOI: 10.1007/s00240-006-0074-0 Epub 2006 Dec 12

[39] Clayman RV, Patel RM, Pearle M. "STONE TREES": Metabolic evaluation and medical treatment of the Urolithiasis patient made easy. Journal of Endourology. 2018;**32**(5):387-392. DOI: 10.1089/end.2017.0541

[40] Skubisz M, Torzewska A, Mielniczek-Brzóska E, Prywer J. Consumption of soft drinks rich in phosphoric acid versus struvite crystallization from artificial urine. Scientific Reports. 2022;**12**(1):14332. DOI: 10.1038/s41598-022-18357-8

[41] Sorensen MD, Harper JD, Borofsky MS, Hameed TA, Smoot KJ, Burke BH, et al. Removal of small, asymptomatic kidney stones and incidence of relapse. The New England Journal of Medicine. 2022;**387**(6):506-513. DOI: 10.1056/NEJMoa2204253

[42] Ratkalkar VN, Kleinman JG. Mechanisms of stone formation. Clinical Reviews in Bone and Mineral Metabolism. 2011;**9**:187-197

[43] Asplin JR, Parks JH, Coe FL. Dependence of upper limit of metastability on supersaturation in nephrolithiasis. Kidney International. 1997;**52**(6):1602-1608

[44] Khan S. Calcium oxalate crystal interaction with renal tubular epithelium, mechanism of crystal adhesion and its impact on stone development. Urological Research. 1995;**23**:71-79

[45] Sorensen MD, Kahn AJ, Reiner AP, Tseng TY, Shikany JM, Wallace RB, et al. Impact of nutritional factors on incident kidney stone formation: A report from the WHI OS. The Journal of Urology. 2012;**187**(5):1645-1649. DOI: 10.1016/j.juro.2011.12.077 Epub 2012 Mar 14

[46] Rodgers A, Gauvin D, Edeh S, Allie-Hamdulay S, Jackson G, Lieske JC. Sulfate but not thiosulfate reduces calculated and measured urinary ionized calcium and supersaturation: Implications for the treatment of calcium renal stones. PLoS One. 2014;**9**(7):e103602. DOI: 10.1371/journal.pone.0103602

[47] Sarica K, İnal Y, Erturhan S, Yağci F. The effect of calcium channel blockers on stone regrowth and recurrence after shock wave lithotripsy. Urological research. 2006;**34**:184-189

[48] Fink HA, Wilt TJ, Eidman KE, Garimella PS, MacDonald R, Rutks IR, et al. Medical management to prevent recurrent nephrolithiasis in adults: A systematic review for an American College of Physicians Clinical Guideline. Annals of internal medicine. 2013;**158**(7):535-543

[49] Hesse A. Urinary Stones: Diagnosis, Treatment, and Prevention of Recurrence. Basel, Switzerland: Karger Medical and Scientific Publishers; 2009

[50] Fink HA, Akornor JW, Garimella PS, MacDonald R, Cutting A, Rutks IR, et al. Diet, fluid, or supplements for secondary prevention of nephrolithiasis: A systematic review and meta-analysis of randomized trials. European urology. 2009;**56**(1):72-80

[51] Siener R, Ebert D, Nicolay C, Hesse A. Dietary risk factors for hyperoxaluria in calcium oxalate stone formers. Kidney international. 2003;**63**(3):1037-1043

[52] Ferraro PM, Taylor EN, Gambaro G, Curhan GC. Soda and other beverages and the risk of kidney stones. Clinical Journal of the American Society of Nephrology. 2013;**8**(8):1389-1395

[53] Siener R. Nutrition and kidney stone disease. Nutrients. 2021;**13**(6):1917. DOI: 10.3390/nu13061917

[54] Hamm LL, Hering-Smith KS. Pathophysiology of hypocitraturic nephrolithiasis. Endocrinology and Metabolism Clinics. 2002;**31**(4):885-893

[55] Ferraro PM, Mandel EI, Curhan GC, Gambaro G, Taylor EN. Dietary protein and potassium, diet–dependent net acid load, and risk of incident kidney stones. Clinical Journal of the American Society of Nephrology. 2016;**11**(10):1834-1844

[56] Siener R, Seidler A, Voss S, Hesse A. The oxalate content of fruit and vegetable juices, nectars and drinks. Journal of Food Composition and Analysis. 2016;**45**:108-112

[57] Hönow R, Hesse A. Comparison of extraction methods for the determination of soluble and total oxalate in foods by HPLC-enzyme-reactor. Food Chemistry. 2002;**78**(4):511-521

[58] Lemann J Jr, Pleuss JA, Worcester EM, Hornick L, Schrab D, Hoffmann RG. Urinary oxalate excretion increases with body size and decreases with increasing dietary calcium intake among healthy adults. Kidney international. 1996;**49**(1):200-208

[59] Taylor EN, Stampfer MJ, Mount DB, Curhan GC. DASH-style diet and 24-hour urine composition. Clinical Journal of the American Society of Nephrology. 2010;**5**(12):2315-2322